"This book is rich with highly usef
that can help you and your child s   _.stablishing a more
peaceful and loving relationship."
—Russell A. Barkley Ph.D., author of *Taking Charge of ADHD*

"Speaking from years of practical experience Taylor-Klaus dispenses
wit, wisdom and effective strategies."
—Sam Goldstein Ph.D., co-author of *Raising Resilient Children*

"Deftly written with humor and compassion, this book offers a
framework for developing a collaborative approach in working with
your child, opportunities for self-reflection, and action-oriented
solutions to some of life's most difficult parent-child issues. This book
is a life saver for many struggling parents who may feel they are barely
holding on."
—Mary Anne Richey, M.Ed., co-author of *Raising Boys with ADHD*

"With wit and wisdom that can only come from experience, Elaine
Taylor-Klaus reminds fellow parents that they really can make a
difference in the lives of their complex kids."
—Susan Stiffelman, MFT, author of *Parenting Without Power Struggles*

"My favorite parenting book, bar none! Raising complex kids is tough
and Taylor-Klaus nails it. A 'must-read' lifeline for parents of struggling
kids. This book will transform your life."
—Melissa Orlov, author of *The ADHD Effect on Marriage*

"This book is smart, engaging, and written for busy (and sometimes
chaotic) families. It teaches parents to use reflection and self-care
to connect with the radical acceptance and the "bring it on" attitude
needed to take on parenting challenges."
—Lidia Zylowska MD, author of *The Mindfulness Prescription for Adult ADHD*

CONTENTS

The Essential Guide to Raising Complex Kids

with ADHD, Anxiety, and More

What Parents and Teachers *Really* Need
to Know to Empower Complicated Kids
with Confidence and Calm

Elaine Taylor-Klaus, PCC, CPCC

To my parents, who encouraged me to pursue a life of purpose and supported me wholeheartedly as I endeavored to raise my complex family with consciousness and grace.

To my collaborator, Diane, whose partnership has made this possible, and to our amazing tribe of parents who inspire me everyday.

To my kids (my puppies) Bex (& Alicia), Syd, and Josh, who have been my greatest teachers.

And to my partner, David, who always believes in me, even when I find it hard to believe in myself.

——

PART 3
Turning Information into Action
Making This Work in Your Life
150

Foreword

"The situation doesn't call for blame or punishment; it calls for understanding and compassion." —Thich Nhat Hanh

Full disclosure: I've known Elaine Taylor-Klaus for years, and I like and respect her very much. So I was not impartial when I opened the pages of this book. I really wanted to like what I read. After all, having agreed to write this foreword, it would have been awkward to have to find an excuse not to write it.

To my delight, the book proved to be even better than I hoped it would be, at least in my estimation, that is. I don't know about your estimation, of course, because I don't know you.

But, since you picked up this book—maybe even bought it—I can make a pretty good guess as to who you are. Likely, you're a mom. Maybe a dad, but more moms read books like this than dads (which is too bad—not that moms read them, of course, but that more dads don't!). And likely you have at least one child you're worried about and want to understand better, as well as better serve.

Of course, you might also be a teacher (I love teachers. My dad was a grade-school teacher, and teachers saved my life all along the way. So if you're a teacher, here's a huge thank you from me!); you might be a grandparent (a close male friend of mine recently told me, "Being a grandparent is the only part of life that isn't overrated"; I'm not a grandparent yet, but I look forward to being one some day); you might be a parent in the making, or a sibling of a complex kid, or maybe you were once a complex kid yourself. Who knows, you might just be someone who picked up this book by chance in a waiting room in Kansas.

But whoever and wherever you are, read on. This is a book that emerges triumphantly and with dignity out of suffering. Elaine has done the hard part. With a glimmer of hope following a difficult decade of parenting, she had what she calls her "Scarlett O'Hara moment" while sitting by herself on a cabin porch in the woods. She stood up, shook her fist at the sky, and said to herself, "As God is my witness, no parent should ever have to go through alone what I did those first ten years."

With this book, she makes good on her promise. The ideas and methods she developed and describes in this book are what she needed to know, and I suspect they're what you need to know too.

I watched this book grow over years. Elaine took great care to get it all right. She put in the sweat and tears required to make a book good. Books don't just happen. Especially if you write them yourself (I know, having written quite a few), they grow fitfully, have to be trimmed and cut, fed and watered, fertilized, and let lie fallow until finally—if you're lucky—the moment of harvest arrives.

Elaine has harvested a magnificent book. Chock-full of practical ideas and solutions, teeming with hard-earned nuggets of wisdom, always a friend to the reader but never a lecturer or preacher, this book will live for many years to come, helping all who read it and sparing those who do (as well as those they love and care for) the unnecessary suffering that lack of understanding, knowledge, and skill always inflict.

So reader, relish and enjoy! Take the knowledge and wisdom in these pages, so engagingly presented, and incorporate them into your daily life; practice the principles, share with others the same, and watch your world and the world of all you touch, from your own children outward, bask in the benefits and grow strong.

—Edward Hallowell, M.D., author of *Driven to Distraction* and
   The Childhood Roots of Adult Happiness

An Introduction for Busy Parents and Professionals

"If, however, we are preoccupied with the fear and despair in us, we can't help remove the suffering of others." —THICH NHAT HANH

You Are Not Alone

On the surface, the first decade of my adult family life looked ideal: a loving marriage; three bright, beautiful children; a nice home; a strong community; good friends; and a close family. If Facebook had been around back then, it would have appeared picture perfect—to the outside world.

On the inside, things always felt on the verge of collapse. My loving, playful husband was inattentive to the family, hyperfocused on his business to an unhealthy extent. My children were missing typical milestones (basic scissor use at age 3, introductory reading at age 5), and every teacher conference was a potential minefield. My friends gave me guilt-inducing advice starting with, "If you would just . . . ," without understanding the challenges I was facing. Frankly neither did I.

When my youngest child was recommended for evaluation at the ripe old age of 4, his older siblings were already being treated for multiple issues. I wondered, "Is my husband really responsible for all of this neurology?" I asked my child's psychiatrist if I might have issues that would explain why I was struggling too. She said, "No honey, you're just a mom."

Being "just a mom" to complex kids turned out to be the most difficult job of my life. Nothing I had ever done or learned prepared me for the challenges—lives filled with therapists, specialists, tutors, school accommodations, special education programs, and so much more. I spent the first decade of parenthood fumbling through the darkness, isolated and alone (despite being in a loving marriage).

Around age 40, I finally had myself evaluated and discovered undiagnosed learning and attention issues. Suddenly, my whole life made sense.

Surrounded by loving family and friends and supportive schools and providers, I had spent more than a decade lost, scared, and confused, alternating between denial and decisive action. I tackled the "problems," but never really understood the big picture of what it meant to be raising "complex kids." As pieces slowly fell into place, propelled by nutritional changes and the addition of coaching for me, life began to transform—for the whole family.

And then, I had my Scarlett O'Hara moment. I was camping, alone on a cabin porch, marveling at how things had improved in such a short time. I looked up to the sky, raised my fist, and said aloud to myself, "As God is my witness, no parent should ever have to go through alone what I did those first 10 years." In time, I realized a deeper truth: no parent *or child* should ever have to go through what *my kids and I* did those first

> We can't eliminate our kids' complex issues (though heaven knows I tried), but I'm here to tell you this: we can damn sure help them learn to manage their issues.

ten years. Or what my husband faced in his childhood and into adulthood. Or what I, my siblings, or my friends did. Something had to change—*for all of us.*

As you no doubt already know, parenting complex kids is not for the faint of heart. Frankly, being a complex kid is no picnic, either. But it doesn't have to be so isolating, overwhelming, confusing, or scary. We can't eliminate our kids' complex issues (though heaven knows I tried), but I'm here to tell you this: we can damn sure help them learn to manage their issues.

We Are More the Same Than We Are Different

Every week, parents I've never spoken with before open their hearts to me. They are the parents of all kinds of complex kids, of all ages, from all over the world. They call or video chat me for "Sanity Sessions." I listen, hear their stories, acknowledge their experiences—and let them know how we can help them help their kids or refer them to someone who can.

I love this part of my work, and I take my responsibility seriously. Their kids are complicated, struggling to hit typical milestones in life and in learning. Many parents have never had a chance to tell their story, or they feel like no one in their lives wants to listen. They describe the wide array of challenges their kids are facing, such as ADHD, anxiety, learning disabilities, depression, ODD, autism, and so much more. And they share frustrations and fears that their kids will not lead independent, successful, or fulfilling lives.

Parents confide in me: They know there's more they could be doing, if only they knew how; sometimes they don't like their kids or don't enjoy parenting; they've already done so much to support their child, and it has cost them dearly, both financially and emotionally.

And, heartbroken, they tell me that nothing seems to have made much of a difference up until now.

And you know what?

No matter how old the parents or grandparents are, how old their kids, where they live in the world, their level of education, or their socioeconomic condition—truly, no matter how different they are from each other—they have more in common than all of their differences combined. Sometimes, they all feel isolated and judged.

Frustrated by tension in the family or worried for their child's future, they tend to want the same things (besides asking me to come live in their house for a few months!). They want:

- a sense of peace and confidence.
- to improve their family's relationships.
- to know that their kid is going to be okay.

They want a clear path, a how-to manual, so they can do the best job possible as parents.

This book is designed to be that interactive how-to manual. It's for parents of complex kids and the professionals serving their families. It doesn't delve into extensive details about any particular childhood condition, *per se*; instead, it fills the gaps, offering a playbook for any adult looking to support the complex kids who need their care.

Drawing from the foundational principles of professional coaching and change management, we'll explore the steps of the Impact Model, which I developed together with my business partner in ImpactParents®, Diane Dempster. With this simple and profoundly effective approach to problem-solving, you'll immediately apply key concepts and fundamental strategies to daily life, ultimately creating lasting change. Before you know it, you'll be parenting or teaching like a coach—and rediscovering the joy of raising complex kids.

Do You Have to Read the Whole Book?

This book walks you through a simple method for parent management in a way that's easy to process and remember, weaving essential concepts and strategies into every section. The short, digestible sections make it easy to process. I'd like you to start from the beginning and read to the end because you'll uncover something new and immediately useful with the turn of every page.

But realistically, it's highly unlikely that everyone will read the book cover to cover. I don't take that personally. How you use this book—as with everything in life—is up to you. Just as there's no one way to raise a complex kid, there's no one way to read this book. Certainly, you'll get the most out of it if you read it all the way through, but I want to give you permission to read it how it serves you best.

How you process information, how you invest your time, how worried you are, your intentions, your motivation, and your follow-through will determine how you use this book. Maybe you will:

- Start from the beginning and find immense value, then perhaps get distracted as your life starts to improve.
- Start with a chapter that appeals to you and seems like a quick fix (or an easy win).
- Start with quotes, images, or subheadings.
- Just read the strategies section in each chapter.
- Read the whole thing.

So, let me offer you a little cheat sheet highlighting what the sections or chapters will provide, so you can identify what's most important for you. As you decide what to read, you'll practice the Impact Action Model:

1. Decide what's important.
2. Gather information.
3. Set a plan.
4. Take action.
5. Expect changes to the plan, modify it, and then try again.
6. Take care of yourself in the process.

Sound like a recipe for managing life?

The Three Parts of the Book

Part One (Chapters 1–4): Covers your role in handling key issues facing your kids, so you can guide them on their path to independence. Whether your child has brain-based issues (such as ADHD, anxiety, learning disabilities, sensory processing, oppositional defiant disorder [ODD], autism, bipolar, attachment, depression, Tourette syndrome, etc.) or metabolic issues (such as juvenile diabetes, celiac disease, food allergies, etc.), they are complex because of a chronic medical condition (or several) children need to learn to manage for themselves in order to ultimately be successful in life.

Part Two (Chapters 5–10): Explains how to use each step of the Impact Model in real life, with specific examples and strategies. Chapters 6, 7, and 8 differentiate this method from other parenting paradigms.

Part Three (Chapters 11–12): Provides a guide to taking action, evaluating, and modifying. It's unreasonable to expect that everything you try will work right away, so you'll learn strategies to tweak efforts and improve outcomes.

The Sections of Each Chapter

Storytelling: Although this quick story may not describe your particular experience, it captures the essence of something familiar, providing a foundational framework for the chapter.

Stating the Problem: Getting clear on the "problem" you're trying to solve is an often overlooked but essential component of problem-solving and creating lasting change.

Coach's Reframe: A coaching perspective for each problem reveals new possibilities for action. Changing perspectives influences outcomes.

Recommended Strategy: Based on the problem and the reframe, this is a tangible strategy to implement immediately.

TAKING A STAND FOR *YOUR* SELF-CARE

Imagine this: You're rafting down a river with your family, when a section of whitewater rapids throws you into the water. There's no time for panic—you've got to hustle. Your kids need you in the boat; besides, it's cold and dangerous in the water! The sooner you get back onto the raft, the better. You reach out your hand so the rafting guide can pull you back on board.

Or do you?

As parents, when something throws us off balance, we have a strange tendency to resist help that gets us back on track. It's as if we're so concerned about our kids staying on the boat that we don't take the hand that's offered to us. Instead we stay in the river, barely treading water behind the raft, which will do nothing to help our kids dodge the next set of rapids downstream.

We've got to prioritize taking care of ourselves and accepting the help we need so we're not left watching helplessly as our kids float out of our reach.

Say No: You can let go of old ideas, patterns, or behaviors to improve the effectiveness of the strategy.

Say Yes: You can add to (or keep in) your repertoire to enhance effectiveness and set yourself up for success.

Self-Talk for Self-Care: Helpful, encouraging mindsets to improve self-care instead of adding to your to-do list.

Questions for Self-Discovery: I strongly encourage you to start a journal so these powerful questions can extend and guide your self-discovery long after you close the book.

A Word about Language

Language can be a powerful tool for effective communication. It can also be used (or perceived) as a weapon of destruction. Sometimes the difference between the two is a thin line. Throughout this book, I'll be very specific about language:

- Sometimes I'll suggest how you might say things to make it easier for kids (or coparents or teachers) to hear.
- I'll caution about certain words or expressions that tend to trigger defensive reactions.
- I'll raise your awareness of the power of words and tone, encouraging you to use them to build connection in your most precious, important relationships.
- I'll warn of the unintended impact you can have when you don't think carefully about what you say and how you say it.

Gender-Inclusive Pronouns

As our kids mature, they continue to ask new things of us as parents. In 2018, my eldest came out as nonbinary and asked me to start using the gender-inclusive pronoun "they." To be candid, as a writer, I find the language awkward, so it's been a difficult transition. Mostly I'm just not accustomed to it yet.

To honor my child's shift in pronouns—and to practice so it becomes more natural—I use the singular they more often than the traditional he or she throughout this book. I hope you'll grant me some grace as I make the effort to meet my kid where they are. I'm committed to staying with it until I am as comfortable with it as their generation (thankfully) seems to be.

Who Is This Book Really For?

Although the stories and examples are generally directed to parents, the methodology is every bit as instructive for other professionals who work with students and their families—including teachers, tutors, therapists, counselors, clinical providers, and in-home behaviorists. Any adult can use a coach approach to enroll young people to take ownership of their lives.

Finally this book is also relevant for adults who are facing challenging conditions themselves. Many of us never learned to understand and manage anxiety, ADHD, or whatever else makes life difficult as adults. So (almost) everything offered in this book is equally applicable to adults. If you want to embrace your unique complications in life and learn to become your best self, you can use this method to manage yourself too. It works for me, my husband, my young adult kids, and thousands of our members and clients around the globe—every day.

Questions for Self-Discovery

- What do you hope this book will help you achieve?
- Which parts interest you? Which chapters?
- Which sections in each chapter appeal to you most?
- What's important about changing your language and your tone?
- How do you resist taking care of yourself?
- Who do you want to help by reading this book? (Hint: this could be a trick question.)

Turning Chaos into Calm

EMBRACING A FAMILY LIFE THAT'S
PERFECTLY IMPERFECT

Do You Have a Complex Kid?

Most parents weather occasional storms. That's life, after all. But with complex children—kids who struggle with life or learning—it can feel like we are living in a constant state of high alert, with a hurricane threatening to move in at any moment.

It's deceptive: The skies appear sunny and blue. But you see that gray cloud looming, closer than you'd like, and you never know when it's going to swoop in and rain on your parade. You never know when your child's challenges are going to hijack family life.

If you're often walking on eggshells or waiting for the other shoe to drop, then you, like me, might have complex kids.

- Are you concerned your child is lazy or disrespectful?
- Do you feel helpless watching your child suffer?
- Does your kid lash out in ugly ways, only to apologize later with deep regret?
- Does your child struggle to make and keep friends?
- Are sibling squabbles much worse than you ever imagined?

- Does your smart kid think they're "stupid" and struggle in school?
- Do you regularly disagree with your coparent about how to help your kid?
- Are you convinced *something's* going on, but your child hasn't been assessed?
- Has your child been diagnosed with a chronic condition?

Maybe your child's been diagnosed with ADHD, learning disabilities, anxiety, depression, autism, sensory processing, food allergies, or something related. Maybe not.

Chances are, there's a reason for their difficult behavior. If you feel like you just don't know how to help your child, or you've tried everything and nothing works, then you are in the right place.

The first part of this book will demystify what's really involved with parenting a complex kiddo. So, I want to invite you to take a deep breath and let it out really slowly. And again. Lengthen your exhale. Now, let's begin.

If you feel like you just don't know how to help your child, or if you've tried everything and nothing works, then you are in the right place.

SARAH'S STORY

Sarah wanted nothing more than to have a family, and it didn't happen as easily as she expected. She and her spouse, Jake, were grateful beyond measure for two healthy children, so it took several years for her to admit that there was trouble in paradise. By age 8, their oldest child was quirky and emotionally sensitive, and their 5-year-old was following a similar path (though possibly mirroring her brother). Concerned, Sarah spent considerable time searching for help. Jake thought Sarah was overreacting, coddling their kids, and being too soft. They had very different approaches to the situation, and their marriage was experiencing a friction they never expected. The more Sarah sought help, the greater Jake's insistence on using a firmer hand. Sarah's resentment grew. She desperately wanted them to be on the same page but couldn't see a path to that happening.

Bottom Line: It took several years for Sarah to admit that there was trouble in paradise.

CHAPTER 1

"This Kid Is Really Smart, but . . ."

Six Challenge Areas for Families with Complex Kids

"Some of the situations and accidents that cause us the greatest suffering, when seen objectively, do not look very big. But because we don't know how to manage them, they feel enormous." —THICH NHAT HANH

Six Key Challenge Areas

Your child is struggling, and so are you. The problems you encounter every day are staggering; the stories range from comical to terrifying. And the challenges you face affect every aspect of family life.

In the creation of ImpactParents.com, Diane and I have found it helpful to categorize this wide range of challenges into six key areas. Families can be impacted in one area, a few, or all six. Consider the *idea* of each category to get a sense of whether it's a familiar challenge for your family.

CHALLENGE AREA 1: EMOTION MANAGEMENT

Whether our kids are quick to anger, painfully shy, surprisingly silly, rule-following and serious, quick to brush things off, or given to taking things personally, they may be struggling with emotional management. Maybe their highs are higher and their lows are lower than their typical peers. Maybe they fly off the handle when things don't go their way or when they hear the word "no." Or maybe they can't handle it when others don't follow "the rules." Regardless, they struggle with emotional self-regulation.

CHALLENGE AREA 2: ORGANIZATION

Your child leaves a trail behind them but doesn't seem to notice. They don't put things away and are oblivious to clutter. They struggle with planning, prioritizing, time management, and/or procrastination. Their room is a wreck; their backpack is overflowing. They don't follow directions well and are constantly losing or forgetting things. They struggle to manage possessions and to take care of their responsibilities.

CHALLENGE AREA 3: HOME/SCHOOL

Your child is intelligent (maybe even gifted), but still struggles with school. They're not reaching their potential, despite all efforts to help them get organized. School reports consistently say they could do better if only they would just "try harder," pay attention, apply themselves, or turn in their work. As if that were easy. They may do homework but forget to turn it in, or they may forget or actually do the wrong assignments. They avoid getting started, ask for last-minute help, or dread projects. They struggle to manage what's expected of them.

CHALLENGE AREA 4: LOGISTICS

Mornings, weekday afternoons, weekends, bedtime, and (sometimes) school breaks are harder than you think they should be. Basic routines seem impossible to do consistently. Your child requires constant reminders to stay on task or do anything. Despite frequent reminders, they don't think sequentially or remember to use systems you've created. Getting them off technology is impossible, and reward systems rarely work for long (if at all). Your child struggles to use simple processes to help life run more smoothly.

CHALLENGE AREA 5: RELATIONSHIPS

Tensions are high at home, and explosions are not uncommon (from kids or parents). You worry your child doesn't know how to make or keep friends. They may have a hard time relating to family members who don't understand them. You disagree with your coparent about how best to support your child, and maybe your marriage suffers under the pressure. Babysitters can't handle your kids. You love your kids, but sometimes you or your spouse check out because you don't feel connected. Your child struggles with relationships.

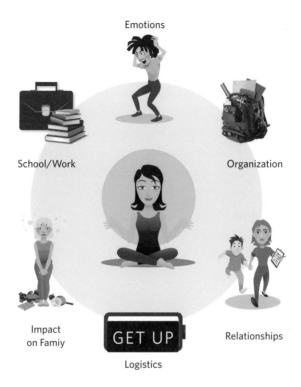

CHALLENGE AREA 6: IMPACT ON THE FAMILY (PARENTS OR SIBLINGS)

This is not what you expected when you became a parent, and you keep waiting for things to get better. Who thought parenting would be this hard? You feel frustrated, disappointed, sad, embarrassed, guilty, and/or aggravated. You're exhausted. Sometimes you don't want to go home. You have so much to be grateful for, yet sometimes your guilty secret is that you want it all to go away. You are struggling with raising a complex child.

The clearer you can get about what challenges you're facing, the better you can address them. Throughout this book, we'll do that together, starting with shifting how you're thinking about the problems in your family life. In coaching, we call this *reframing*.

Coach's Reframe: Parent from Inspiration, Not Desperation

In almost every conversation I have with parents of complex kids, I encounter deep love and loyalty. Parents are tenacious. We are passionately committed to our children's success—often at the expense of our own health and wellness.

Parents of complex kids are hard working, diligent, resourceful, engaged—and exhausted, overwhelmed, scared, and doggedly committed.

If we're not careful, we become desperate. In fact, "I'm desperate" is one of the most common phrases I hear on first calls with parents (usually followed by "I just want some peace.").

Desperation is not an effective way to inspire kids to reach their full potential. When we parent from desperation, we focus on what is broken, what's not working, and what we're afraid of. It's a fear-based energy drain, and our kids feel it. If we believe they can, or they can't, we'll end up being correct—and they'll take their lead from us.

When we shift our approach from inspiration to parenting, the possibilities are endless. It's the classic shift from pessimism to optimism, seeing the glass as half full. When I was growing up, one of my brothers was a pessimist, and the other was an optimist. My parents used to say that if the optimist entered a room full of horse poop, he would start shoveling happily, exclaiming, "There's got to be a pony in here somewhere." I wanted to be an "octopus" (aka optimist) like my brother. Even as a young child, I sensed it was a "better" (or at least happier) way to go through life.

> Reframe your mindset to focus on what's possible for your child.

It's tempting to focus on what's wrong and allow that to dominate your responses. But that makes it easy to get discouraged too. So, I want to encourage you to use the challenge areas to clarify *what you want to see improved*, reframe your mindset, and focus on what's possible for your child.

My job in this book is to help you step out of desperation, so you can feel inspired by what's possible for your kids, by their capacity to grow to become amazing adults. And I want to guide you to see, and to truly believe, that you are uniquely equipped to help them get there!

To inspire kids to believe in themselves, you'll want to shed yourself of desperation. That doesn't mean taking a Pollyanna approach to their challenges or pretending they don't exist. Quite the opposite. It means you'll begin to view the obstacles practically, without the baggage of shame, blame, and fear. Then you can navigate them deftly with confidence and calm.

Personally, I learned to thread the needle between my two brothers: I became a practical optimist. I see challenges for what they are and choose to start searching for that pony. And you can too. Whether you seek better information to demystify your child's challenges, insight into what other parents

A CASE STUDY IN REFRAMING

A client offered this reframe, and gave me permission to share it:

"I had an epiphany today. I realized my son's ADHD has been a weight around my neck. But it's not all bad. And I forget that. There are many awesome things about ADHD. It seems my brain and heart gravitate toward the negative and forget to integrate the positive. So I choose to reframe! Here is my Reframing List:

- Trouble paying attention → Flexible thinking
- Hyperactive → Spontaneous
- Impulsive → Creative and inventive
- Hyperfocused → A positive superpower
- Distracted → Sees changes in surroundings that others miss
- Emotional dysregulation → Straightforward expression of emotions
- Distractible → Curious
- Intrusive → Eager
- Can't stay on point → Sees connections others miss
- Forgetful → Involved in what he's doing
- Disorganized → Spontaneous
- Stubborn → Persistent
- Moody → Sensitive"

experience, or new ways to tackle old problems, you are not alone. There is hope and possibility ahead for you and your kids. As you let go of desperation, you'll discover the power of inspiration for yourself, ultimately empowering your kids to discover their own path to their greatest potential.

Strategy: Shed the Shoulds

Before we become parents, we have expectations for what kind of parent we'll be and what kind of child we'll have. We imagine our partners as parents and how we'll be as a family. And then, we start noticing the expectations of the outside world—the ones from parents, in-laws, siblings, neighbors, and friends. They come from media, midwives, doulas, doctors, pregnancy books, and classes. And eventually they'll also come from teachers and professionals in our kids' schools and lives.

Before we know it, we're living in an impossible matrix of other people's expectations. Their "shoulds" disconnect us from what we really want for our kids, our families, and ourselves. We start operating on "expectations auto-pilot," trying to fulfill everybody else's vision of what we "should" do.

We end up "shoulding" all over everyone, believing our kids should:

- Sleep through the night by the time they're 4 months old;
- Learn to read before kindergarten;
- Eat five fruits and vegetables daily;
- Eat no artificial sugar;
- Follow our directions (the first time, every time);
- Always speak respectfully;
- Do schoolwork without complaining;
- Not fight with their siblings;
- Make friends easily; or
- Not be shy, hyperactive, or bossy.

The list continues. It starts with the pregnancy police (judging every morsel you eat, your work hours, and your travel schedule); the IVF monitors (who tell you to "just relax"); and the adoption agencies (that ask for extensive references and guarantees). It continues with decisions around feeding, medical care, and schooling . . . and it will continue unabatedly until you realize something: You can't raise this child for everyone else.

Because we internalize the "should" and convince ourselves it's what "good" parents do, we don't realize how much energy we spend fulfilling everyone else's expectations. You (rightfully) want to be seen as a good parent, but in the process, are you losing sight of what's most important to you?

Are you "shoulding" all over yourself?

- **Notice your language.** Beware of obligatory words such as *must, need to, gotta, ought to, have to,* and *should.*

- **Notice how feelings lead to actions.** Beware doing something out of embarrassment or shame or to influence what others think about you or your child.
- **Notice your child.** Beware them covering up challenges or problems to look like they're a "good kid."

To shed the should:

- **Identify the source of each "should."** Is it coming from what you think is important? Or someone/somewhere else?
- **Decide if it's true for you.** Ask yourself, "What's important to me about this?"
- **Change your language.** Replace the obligatory "should" words with "want to," "get to," or "choose to." Notice how that changes your thoughts and feelings.

Once you understand your "shoulds," you'll find dozens of strategies throughout this book to help you shed them. I also encourage you to get to know your values, which are a reflection of what's important to you, what you stand for, and what gives your life meaning. If you need somewhere to start, try https://impactparents.com/parents-clarifying-values/. Your values are your best guide to making decisions based on what's most important to you as a parent—and a powerful way to "shed the shoulds."

Say No to Holding onto Resentment

In the blog post "Parenting Together: Getting on the Same Page," my husband David Taylor-Klaus (DTKCoaching.com) writes:

"Imaginary conversations killed our marriage—almost. During our first decade as parents, so many of the 'conversations' Elaine and I had about expectations around parenting were imaginary . . . When one parent feels like s/he is doing it alone, resentment builds. Communication grinds to a halt. Co-parenting relationships crumble because of the **unspoken**, rather than because of the **spoken**."

When things don't go how you think they should, you'll look for a reason for your disappointment. And when you feel like something isn't fair—maybe that your child is struggling with challenges, or that too much of the burden of handling them falls on you—resentment finds its foothold.

Sometimes we resent others—our partners, other parents, teachers, even our friends—because we feel that they don't understand our urgent need to help our kids. Other times, we do it to ourselves, giving so much to our kids without taking care of ourselves that we end up giving ourselves away. Eventually we become resentful or guilty.

Resentment blossoms in silences and can build quickly. It halts effective communication, putting up barriers to connection and intimacy. It leads to judgment and blame, taking things personally, and feeling put-upon. But resentment withers away in the face of open communication.

"Many things changed over a period of many years, but what's clear to us now is that we never gave up on each other or on the family we wanted to create with each other. Elaine never gave up on me, even when we weren't on the same page. Elaine trusted that my intentions were good. Over time, as she learned more about ADHD, she found ways to share her learning with me despite my defensiveness. We began to have conversations with less judgment, less resentment, and more acceptance of each other and our kids."

The biggest challenge to letting go of resentment is that we hold onto it because we feel justified. Resentment feels easier than having difficult conversations. It feels safer than sharing our truths or expressing what we really want for ourselves and our kids. Letting go of resentment without blaming or feeling blamed requires vulnerability, which isn't easy for any of us.

David ended his article with this challenge to parents: "Start a new conversation. Ask what's important to your co-parent. LISTEN. Get curious. Don't make any major decisions. Just explore each other's perspectives and look for commonality."

When you feel unfairly treated, you may have good reason to feel resentful. Frankly, it's likely that things aren't fair. But remember, resentment festers and destroys, preventing you from being the kind of parent you really want to be. It's up to you to stop holding it tightly. Resentment is yours to let go. I know it's not easy to do, but I assure you it's worth the effort.

Say Yes to Acceptance

My oldest child always marched to the beat of their own drum. Frankly, they were rockin' out to an entirely different orchestra. Even though I firmly believed it was good for them to dance to their own music, sometimes it was hard to keep dancing myself. Candidly, I had no clue what music was playing much of the time!

Over the years, I found myself a little lost with each of their childhood milestones. I was out of sync with my friends and sometimes a little jealous. It was hard to find my place among my peers when my child was on such a different path. Sometimes, I learned to take it in stride. Other times their "differences" would hit me like a ton of bricks.

Their high school graduation was a great example. For years I had an image of watching my kid cross the stage at Symphony Hall on graduation day. Instead, they graduated at another school, in another state, with a class of fifteen kids in a "2E" school for twice exceptional kids, both gifted and challenged.

We attended the lovely backyard-style graduation, surrounded by parents we didn't know. While I felt like a guest at my own wedding, I had more in common with these parents than I realized. Though they didn't know us at all, these parents understood our journey and what it meant to raise an intensely bright, complicated child. They understood the challenges of educating a child for whom "doing school" did not come naturally.

> At some point all parents need to modify expectations to meet the child they have, not the child they thought they'd have.

In addition to earning a hard-won high school diploma, my teen reached a major milestone with their peers. They marched in a cap and gown—and floral-lined combat boots. Their successes, both in and out of school, were acknowledged and celebrated. I sat gratified to revel with my peers.

I've grown to accept and embrace my child's path in life. And when I find myself standing on the sidelines of a game they're no longer playing, I gently remind myself that my child left the field in search of a game better suited for them, and I'm really proud of them for that.

Our lives are enmeshed with our children's lives; our vision for them is intricately tied to our vision for ourselves. When their challenges change the course of their future, it impacts how we see ourselves. Accepting our kids for who they are often means reimagining our dreams for ourselves too.

To effectively support kids in their growth and development, at some point all parents need to modify expectations to meet the child they have, not the child they thought they'd have. As keynoter Ross Greene said at the 2019 International Conference on ADHD, "The most important task for parents: figure out who your child is. Get comfortable with it."

Self-Talk: Expect the Unexpected (Bring It On!)

In a previous life, I taught childbirth yoga classes. I loved helping couples prepare for the physical and emotional challenges of childbirth and the unexpected challenges of postpartum parenting. I learned tremendous pearls of wisdom in those years. The most lasting lesson was a parenting companion to "Man plans, G-d laughs." Simply put, expect the unexpected and be prepared for anything. They are words to live by.

With complex kids, it's reasonable to expect that things won't always go as planned. There will be hiccups along your path that you could never have imagined. Sometimes, they'll throw you off course.

But most of the time, things are not really the crises we make them out to be. Usually, what upsets us most is that things aren't going according to plan. That can feel stressful—for our kids (especially those with anxiety) and for us.

When things don't go smoothly, we can freak out and react, go all gloom and doom, and fight the change. Or we can embrace the unexpected and find the silver lining. In any given upset, there's generally an opportunity to foster resilience and learning. The ability to see things as a possibility rather than a catastrophe is what I call a "Bring it on!" attitude. This guiding principle brought me enormous comfort as a parent.

I want you to learn to trust yourself, to know that—whatever life throws at you—you've got this! You can hit, catch, dodge, whatever it takes. No matter what the surprise—and there will be surprises—you can learn to trust that you are creative and resourceful, and you can handle whatever comes your way.

Eventually, you'll learn to do this with grace, a smile, and maybe even suppressed laughter when your child tries to flush an entire roll of toilet paper at once (true story). Wouldn't you rather laugh than cry in those moments?

HOW TO REMEMBER "YOU'VE GOT THIS!"

Remind yourself that the unexpected is actually to be expected.

Unexpected upsets are legit feelings. When things start to escalate, consciously handle the intense feelings, and teach your kids to do the same. Kids can knock down blocks or scream into pillows when they get mad. Respect intense feelings, and practice recovering from upsets. (See Chapter 2.)

Avoid making your kids feel "wrong" for not having the kind of self-control that you (and they) would like. Help them see that self-management takes time. Shift your thinking. For example:

- If your child is driven by a motor, help them learn to slow themselves down.
- Remember your child needs constant stimulation.
- Accept that self-control develops gradually, one table manner at time.
- Make corrections without judgment so they don't feel embarrassed for not being developmentally ready.

Take aim on staying calm in response to anything unsettling that happens (see Chapter 5). The calmer you are, the better for everyone.

Remind yourself, "I've got this" in moments when you do, so you can believe it in moments when you're not so sure. Lean into your successes. Even if you don't know what to do right away, trust that you'll figure it out.

Remember you are generally a capable adult. For real. When you put your mind to it, you are resourceful, competent, and effective. You don't have to have dealt with something previously to know that you can. Whatever comes around the corner, you've got this!

Questions for Self-Discovery

- Which of the six challenge areas are relatable to you?
- How do you parent from inspiration? From desperation?
- What "should" do you want to let go?
- What resentments are you holding?
- What do you want to accept?
- When will you remind yourself "I've got this"?

JANINE'S STORY

The apple doesn't fall far from the tree. Janine likely has ADHD and anxiety just like her kids, though she's never been diagnosed or treated. Before having a family, she'd managed to get through school and do well enough, though she tended to beat herself up for chronic lateness, forgetfulness, or "stupid" mistakes. She married an organized man who was attracted to her lively exuberance. When she became responsible for running the household with three kids, her husband accused her of not trying hard enough. No matter how good things looked on the outside, inside she was frequently on the verge of tears, except when she got angry and lashed out—sometimes at her children, mostly at her spouse and herself. When I suggested she put the stick down and forgive herself so she could start managing her challenges effectively, she cried with relief. It was the first time she ever gave herself credit for what she was doing (against great odds), instead of what she wasn't.

Bottom Line: Janine tended to beat herself up and was frequently on the verge of tears, except when she got angry and lashed out. When I suggested that she put down the stick that she'd been beating herself with for so many years, she cried with relief.

CHAPTER 2

"This Is Not What I Expected"

Parenting Complex Kids Is Different

> "A good environment allows the best things in us to manifest. A toxic environment can bring out the worst things in us." —THICH NHAT HANH

Common (but Unhelpful) Parenting Reactions

When life throws you curveballs, don't keep swinging at the problem without changing your approach. Although there is no single "right" way to parent, there are definitely some approaches that aren't optimal and can even make things more difficult for everyone, including you.

Here are some less than optimal ways that parents typically respond when raising complex kids. Sometimes these approaches work, which is seductive; over time, though, they usually create friction. If you've already put a lot of effort into trying to help your kid—by reading books, going to doctors, maybe even taking a parenting class—this section can give you an understanding of why things haven't worked yet. (You can also try the Parenting Style Quiz at impactparents.com/help-for-parents/parenting-style-quiz/.) The rest of this chapter will offer ways to shift to a new approach.

Angry Ann and Angry Andy: You get angry and lose your temper all too often, even though you don't want to. It's all so frustrating. Whatever you do, it never seems to be enough. You feel like you can't get a break. You say, "I feel like I'm always yelling, but it's not my style."

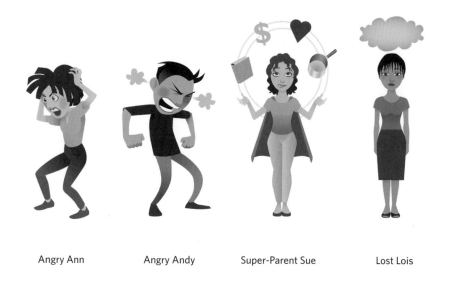

Angry Ann   Angry Andy   Super-Parent Sue   Lost Lois

Super-Parent Sue: You keep the balls in the air. You look like you have things under control, but you're doing too much and it's not sustainable. You want others to step up and do their fair share, but you don't make the time or help them learn how. Secretly, you'd rather do it yourself, though you still complain, "I'm doing it all, but this is just too much!"

Lost Lois: You feel alone, surrounded by people who don't understand what you're going through. You're doing all you can to support your kids, keep your house running smoothly, and manage everyone's needs. You've lost any direction for yourself and feel like you're running in circles. You say, "I don't know what to do. I feel lost and lonely."

A NOTE ON GENDER STEREOTYPES

Angry Ann and Angry Andy are a reminder that we all have many of these tendencies, regardless of gender. Women can be Distant Dans, and men can be Nagging Nans. Because most of us can relate to several of these, don't let gender distract you from identifying your tendencies.

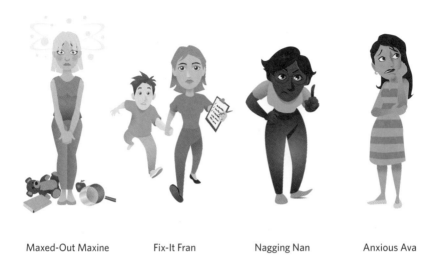

| Maxed-Out Maxine | Fix-It Fran | Nagging Nan | Anxious Ava |

Maxed-Out Maxine: You're overwhelmed and don't know how to handle it anymore. Nothing seems to work, and honestly, you're tired of trying. You want to be a good parent, but sometimes you feel like giving up. You want to do something—*anything*—to make things different! You say, "I'm exhausted. How long can I keep this up?"

Fix-It Fran: You've tried everything imaginable to help your child. You ping-pong from one thing to another, determined to find a solution that works. You see what needs to be done and frequently give your child systems to use (though they rarely do). You say, "I'll do whatever it takes to help my child."

Nagging Nan: You're constantly reminding your kids to do everything they're responsible for and finding things for them to do, just to make sure they're doing something. Your kids are frequently annoyed with you and want you to leave them alone. You say, "If I don't remind them, it won't get done."

Anxious Ava: You're always worried about what isn't getting done or what might go wrong. You catastrophize and fret that you or your coparent are not doing enough as parents. You manage your anxiety by planning and trying to get everyone to follow every little structure you put in place. You say, "I'm worried about what might happen."

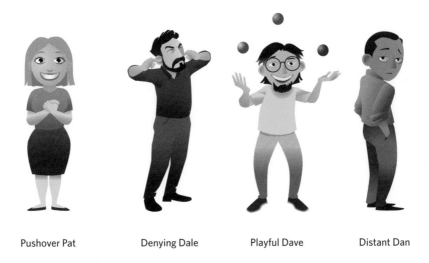

Pushover Pat   Denying Dale   Playful Dave   Distant Dan

Pushover Pat: You're kind and caring. You don't set limits, but when you do, you don't usually follow through with them. You don't like the way family members talk to you, but you don't know how to change it. You just want the family to get along and feel safe, but someone's always upset. You say, "I just want everyone to be happy."

Denying Dale: You have a wait-and-see attitude. You believe that if your child would apply themselves, things would be fine. You're waiting for them to grow out of this stage. You don't want them evaluated because you're concerned about "stigma." You resist a diagnosis because you don't want it used as an excuse for poor behavior. You say, "He must learn to do what he's told."

Playful Dave: You love to play with your kids and are the fun parent. When your spouse (or ex) tries to talk about problems, you don't have much to say—things aren't really that bad. You're glad you don't have to do the "heavy lifting" of parenting, but don't think you get enough credit for keeping things light. You say, "I don't know what you're so worried about."

Distant Dan: You want to be positive, but you're constantly disappointed and you don't feel like you have much say in the matter, anyway. You didn't expect parenting to require so much from you, and sometimes you feel like throwing in the towel. You say, "Why can't they just do what's expected of them?"

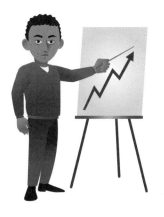
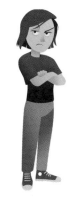
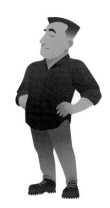

Demanding Randy   Defensive Drew   Bootstrap Bill

Demanding Randy: You have high expectations of your children, setting the bar high so they can't reach their full potential. You accept that your child has challenges but don't want them used as an excuse. You think your coparent is coddling, despite kids needing to overcome challenges to be successful. You say, "You need to do what's expected of you."

Defensive Drew: You care about being a good parent and want others to see you that way. You see kids' respect and obedience as a reflection on you, so you tend to take things personally. If you feel disrespected, you may lash out in blame; if ashamed, you may avoid conflict or embarrassment. You say, "You can't talk to me that way" or, "It's not my fault."

Bootstrap Bill: You didn't have an easy path as a child, but you turned out okay. The school of hard knocks worked for you, and you believe it'll work for your kids too. They need to learn to suck it up and do what's expected of them. Sure, it's hard, but they have to push through and live with disappointment. You say, "Kids have to learn that life isn't fair."

Coach's Reframe: Up Until Now

A number of years ago, I lost a lot of weight. I never went on a diet. I didn't read any books. In fact, after three kids, I had decided to accept my middle-aged body for what it was—about 25 pounds overweight. I decided to stop worrying about my weight.

Instead, I focused on getting healthy, one minor change at a time. After all, what we pay attention to grows (or shrinks, in this case). I lost more than 30 pounds simply by focusing on making healthy choices and choosing to start fresh each day.

Lasting change happens when we shift our perspective and face forward toward the future, focusing on what lies ahead of us, instead of what has happened in the past—up until now. This is true of all kinds of parents.

If you're a neurotypical parent with your executive function skills intact, it can seem mind boggling that others don't approach things as clearly, methodically, or efficiently as you do. You do research, consult experts, and create systems to get things under control; or maybe you double down on discipline.

If you're a complex parent yourself, you've likely been struggling through years of strife, trying to manage everything. It's seriously daunting as you're called upon to make complex medical decisions surrounded by stigma and misinformation (see Chapter 5). Parenting feels like a Jenga game of waiting, expecting all the pieces to come tumbling down.

Either way, when you focus only on what's wrong, it's hard to find a path to something that feels right. It's almost impossible to make sustainable change in life without shifting your underlying thoughts or mindset. And that brings us back to three key words: *Up Until Now.*

There is nothing you can change about anything that has happened in your life up until now. School issues. Relationship dynamics. Arguments. Embarrassing moments. Choices you regret. You can't change anything from the past.

The beauty of this moment is that you have the power to change what happens from here forward. Up until now, you did the best you could with what was available to you. Maybe you tried to get support for your family. Maybe you followed advice from friends, family, and professionals, even if it didn't always get results.

From here, you have an opportunity to start fresh. Armed with the peaceful arsenal of tools and strategies in this book, you can take on a new perspective. You have a chance to try again.

Making choices is what life is all about. Fundamentally, everything is a choice, even when it feels like you don't have one. Every action, every inaction, every conversation started, and every talk avoided is a choice.

Creating change is not just about finding the next action. It's about becoming aware of the choices you're making every day, choices that are influenced by your thoughts and the words you tell yourself.

> The beauty of this moment is that you have the power to change what happens . . . from here forward.

Because you are making choices every moment of every day, the up-until-now perspective can free you up to make decisions that lead to genuine and lasting change. It's based on awareness of the choices you're making, a shift in perspective about what's possible, and the belief that you can influence the circumstances that are causing challenges in your life.

Up until now, change may not have seemed possible; now it's up to you.

Strategy: Consciously Manage Triggers (Four Steps to Escaping the Stress Cycle)

Do you struggle to stay calm when you or someone around you makes a simple (albeit significant) mistake? Is it hard to keep your cool when your kids lose theirs?

We all lose it sometimes. It's human nature to surrender to a meltdown or explosion when pushed past our limit. Sometimes it works to get people's attention, but it's counterproductive, long term.

Overreacting *only* teaches kids that it's okay to go all drama-queen when things don't go their way. When you're upset, how you respond sets the stage for how kids learn to handle upsetting situations. Yelling might get them to do chores, but it won't teach them to take responsibility or manage big emotions. And it definitely makes it harder for them to focus on homework.

When you're at the brink of breaking, it takes Herculean effort to model self-control, to be the "grown-up" when things get triggered. As you learn to keep cool and focus on calming down, it shifts the pattern for everyone in the household.

Here's how you can get started:

FOUR STEPS TO ESCAPING THE STRESS CYCLE

1. **Recognize when someone's brain is triggered.** According to the American Institute of Stress, more than 70 percent of people say they "regularly experience" symptoms "caused by stress," so you likely know what stress feels like. During stress, the primitive brain operates

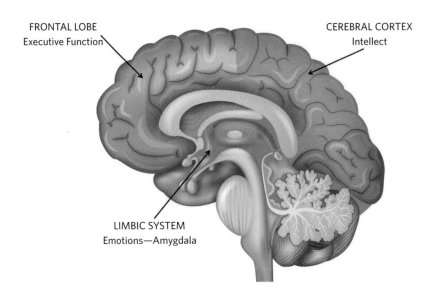

FRONTAL LOBE
Executive Function

CEREBRAL CORTEX
Intellect

LIMBIC SYSTEM
Emotions—Amygdala

as if there's a sabretooth tiger at the cave, taking over the frontal lobe with amygdala hijack, a term that describes a "fight, flight, or freeze" response, coined by Daniel Goleman in his 1995 book *Emotional Intelligence*. This is helpful when avoiding a car accident by hitting the brakes, but not helpful if you get triggered whenever a teacher sends an email. When things get heated, notice if someone's getting triggered (arguing or defensive).

2. **Reclaim the brain from amygdala hijack.** Immediately focus on calming things down and avoid pushing anyone over the edge. Like turning off sirens when you know there's been a false alarm, reclaim the brain by taking deep breaths, taking walks, sipping water, going for a run, watching a funny video, petting the dog, etc. (Yes, sipping water! It sends a message to the primitive brain, as if you were at a watering hole, that it's safe.) This may take time, so beware of "fake calm" (such as three shallow breaths followed by, "Okay, I'm calm now.") Take time to *really* calm down with humor and patience.

3. **Make up a new story that works for you.** The stories we tell ourselves can be harmful or helpful; set us up for failure or success; freak us out or calm us down. Make up a helpful story that you can believe.

For example, thinking "this 7-year-old is a brat," will lead you to treat him like he's purposefully obnoxious. But telling yourself "he's embarrassed" or "this scared little boy needs encouragement" can lead to compassion.

A client's extremely anxious 11-year-old daughter begged to play hockey with the boys, but then resisted going to practice. Her mom felt manipulated; but when asked, "what else is true?" she realized, "The fear is real for her. She's not trying to be difficult. She wants to play, but she's terrified." The new story paved a path to better understanding, connection, and outcomes.

4. **Take action based on the new story.** Once that mom saw a reasonable explanation for her daughter's behavior, they worked together to negotiate attendance at hockey practices, slowly helping her daughter find ways to participate. It was a huge breakthrough.

Escaping the stress cycle can take time to learn to manage, so give yourself some grace in the process. I recall one afternoon when unloading the dishwasher became a huge fight. I was trying to help my child calm down and my husband thought I was letting them off the hook. He struggled with my approach, arguing "It's their job and it needs to get done now." I was between a rock and a hard place. I knew that keeping them from going over the edge was more important than getting the dishes put away, but it was hard to articulate that in a way he could accept. Quietly and calmly I explained, "please trust me; they need to calm down first," removing myself until we could all allow calmer heads to prevail.

Say No to Denial

We knew my eldest was complex starting at two weeks (cholic), then at two years (allergies), then four (learning), then six (emotional). We addressed each health development individually. But to be honest, they were eight (with a list of about 8 diagnoses) before I accepted that they had "special needs." I didn't begin to understand the full impact of what that meant until they were 10 years old.

I thought I was addressing their problems every step of the way. In some ways, I was. There were therapies and doctors and specialists galore. But for many years I was busying myself with the details, missing the big picture.

Swimming deep in the waters of denial, lost in the current, I just kept believing that it was enough that I knew how to swim.

Ever feel like you're stuck in the muddy river of denial? On one level, you know something's going on that needs your attention; on another level, you'd like to pretend it doesn't exist. Most of us begin that way, to be honest. Ideally we start to snap out of it once we realize our kids need our help.

> To guide your kids to safety and success, acknowledge their challenges (and your own) and tackle them head on.

For me, maybe I wanted to make sure things turned out as I had planned—to hold on to my dreams for my child's future (and my own). Maybe I was holding tight because I was afraid to lose control completely. But whatever I was doing clearly wasn't working. It took a decade to understand that to stay true to my larger vision of raising a healthy, independent child, I needed to change my mindset and approach things differently.

SOME SIGNS OF DENIAL

Do you try to protect your kids, thinking things such as

- I don't want the stigma of a "label."
- Maybe it's a phase. I'll wait, hope, and "normalize" life until they grow out of it.
- I won't tell them, so they won't use their diagnosis as an excuse.
- I don't want them to think anything is wrong with them.

Do you try to protect yourself, thinking things such as

- I'm already overwhelmed. I can't handle anything else.
- There's nothing wrong with my child. I'm a good parent.
- I can fix this before it becomes a real problem.
- I'm doing everything the experts suggest, so it will be okay.

To guide your kids to safety and success, it's best to acknowledge their challenges (and your own) and tackle them head on.

Given the challenges our kids face, it's hard enough to guide them to follow their path and develop a vision for themselves. It's nearly impossible when we convince ourselves that there's nothing fundamental that needs to be addressed.

The greatest gift you can give yourself and your complex child, is to acknowledge that whatever issue your child is facing is one of those bumps on your parenting journey that requires course correction. It's not a barrier, but it calls for careful navigation.

You do not have to abandon your goals and dreams when you accept that things aren't going as planned. In fact, hold fast to your dreams! They will serve you and your child extremely well.

But you don't have to stay stuck in the muddy river of denial either. It's scary down there in the muck. When you accept and acknowledge that something's going on that needs your attention, you'll be able to climb out to safety—and get the help you need to steer clear of the obstacles that threaten your child's path, so you can navigate to success.

Say Yes to Forgiveness

It was a Monday morning. I was trying to get the kids moving when I heard my husband shout, "Everyone, get shoes on and get outside—NOW!"

He got my attention. He was calm, but I could tell something was urgent. Wait, why was he even still at home? I called out and he responded, "I've had an ADHD moment and I need some help, please." His voice was strained. Wow. I secretly gave him points for keeping cool, though I was definitely getting nervous!

I went outside to assess the situation. It was like a scene from Stephen King's *Christine*. Two headlights stared out at me from the woods, taunting me. My husband's Prius was halfway down the hill, mere inches from a giant oak tree and our neighbor's wooden fence.

I went back inside to rally the troops. I covered up my white blouse, because things were likely to get messy. I asked everyone to put on closed-toed shoes and long pants—gotta be specific with complex kids. I figured the snakes were already pretty mad.

We came together as a team to push the car out of the woods. It was touch-and-go for a minute, but soon she was out of danger. Within five minutes, the drama was over, everyone was back in their own space, my shirt was clean, and my husband was headed to his meeting. We all handled it like rock stars.

In the world of complex kids, every day feels a little like that Monday morning:

THE 4 STEPS TO ESCAPING THE STRESS CYCLE IN ACTION

When my daughter with ADHD, anxiety, and dyslexia was freaking out about a high school writing assignment, I used this strategy. Keeping my voice as matter-of-factly as possible, I said

Step 1: "Sweetie, can you see that you're getting triggered by this right now?" She nodded, explaining between sobs why everything was so bad. I listened.

Step 2: "What strategies have you used before to calm yourself down?" Sobs. "What if you take a few deep, slow breaths? I'll get you some water. Will you try?" We took time to help her reclaim her brain.

Step 3: "What do you think about this assignment right now?" She responded with a litany of why she couldn't handle it. She vented and I summarized: "You're thinking that you can't do this project." She nodded. "What if that's not actually true? What's another way of looking at this that doesn't feel so stressful?" We explored many options and landed on, "I don't have to write the whole paper tonight, just the thesis statement." That was true, she could believe it, and it was much easier for her to manage.

Step 4: "Now that you see you have to write only a thesis statement to get started, what's the first thing for you to do from here?"

- There is excitement and enthusiasm. Adrenaline is pumping, and we respond to life's adventures with excessive energy. On a good day, we do it with excellent humor as well.
- With unexpected surprises, there can be a serious need for forgiveness. We make simple mistakes a lot—the natural consequence of the marriage of impulsivity and inattention. I know everyone makes mistakes, but we do it bigger, better, and more often.

Striking the balance between jumping to action and managing the agony of defeat is the art of living well with complex kids.

No matter how many strategies we put into place, we're going to have those "ADHD moments." We're going to miss an appointment, forget a school car-pool, or overreact and lose our temper. We're human. When we do, forgiveness (for ourselves and each other) is just as important as responsiveness. Maybe even more.

This story is a classic example: Running late for a meeting, my husband turned on the car in the garage, put it into reverse to back out, and remembered he left something in the house. After running back inside, he returned to find the car halfway across the driveway on its way down the hill. He hadn't heard the Prius, which started to move when the gas engine kicked in. It was an honest mistake.

> You do not have to abandon your goals and dreams when you accept that things aren't going as planned.

Thankfully, and miraculously, no one was hurt; nothing was really damaged except a few scratches and a little pride.

But not a lot of pride. Instead of beating himself up, my husband handled the situation beautifully. He responded quickly, got the help he needed, stayed calm, kept his sense of humor, and let it go when the crisis was past. I'm sure he got a little red in the face when he arrived late to his meeting, but at least he had a great story to tell. He did a masterful job of modeling self-for-giveness for his colleagues and his family.

When mistakes happen—and they will—try to hold them lightly. Practice radical forgiveness. And remember to keep your sense of humor. Who knows, maybe the next car to lurch independently out of the garage will be yours!

Self-Talk: Put the Stick Down

During one summertime family supper, we were eating late, and it was unusu-ally chaotic:

- My middle child wanted one food at a time on her plate.
- My youngest talked incessantly, eating the crumbly chicken topping with his fingers.
- My eldest cracked jokes, entertaining and riling the rest, shoveling in food so fast we wondered if they breathed at all.

There was lively conversation, some mild bickering about who got to talk first, and an equal amount of laughter and playfulness. And there was an unbelievable amount of movement.

I reflected on my childhood, when we ate proper dinners in the dining room, sat up tall in our chairs, and said, "Yes, ma'am" and "Yes, sir" without reminder. Our fingers did not touch the plate. It was interesting—intelligent humor was rewarded—but not exactly lively fun. Formal family dinners had defined my expectations for parenting success.

I had beaten myself up for years because our family's dinners were not "respectable" enough and my household was generally chaotic. That night, looking around, I laughed out loud. My son had climbed onto his sister's back and then returned to his seat for second helpings.

I asked, "Could any of you imagine doing this at Grandpa's house?" Peals of laughter.

In an instant, I appreciated and reveled in the joyous time my family was having. We were loud, rambunctious, and a little wacky, having a blast making memories that foster a lifetime of connection. And I realized that fun is more important to me than propriety.

It was time to put the stick down. I wanted my adult kids to remember connecting, playing, loving, knowing, and accepting each other during family dinners—and I wanted to give myself permission to fully appreciate it. For me, that was success.

Sometimes we make mistakes. We lose our cool, don't handle something as well as we'd like, miss a flight, or forget to pack something important for a trip. Sometimes our kids don't behave as we'd like—bouncing off the walls or melting down. Often, we take these situations personally and beat ourselves up.

But you can reframe self-criticism, bring yourself a little compassion, and practice putting the stick down. Chances are, you've been doing the best you can; and although you can't change the past, your mindset will most assuredly define your future.

Are you going to do everything perfectly from here forward? Nope. But can you imagine how much better you'll do if you stop beating yourself up for whatever might be less than perfect from the past (that is, about a minute ago)?

When the chaos reaches a crescendo, I still get frustrated and long for the reserve of my youth. But that family dinner was a turning point for me.

If my family needs dinnertime to be an aerobic activity, I decided to be okay with that. Although I remain a stickler for "yes, ma'am" (a Southern sign of respect), I've let go of the "shoulds" I beat myself up with for years.

We need to give ourselves permission to have moments of imperfection and handle those moments with grace and a little self-love. When my kids are being their boisterous, creative, funny selves, I want them to feel accepted, not scolded. They're going to need that feeling when they get out there in the big world.

> Chances are, you've been doing the best you can; and although you can't change the past, your mindset will most assuredly define your future.

So I want to encourage you to put the stick down. Beating yourself up is not going to help things get any better and it stands in the way of your enjoying the relationships you have. Whenever you notice that life is slipping out of control, that your well-laid-out plans aren't working, or that you could have handled something better, put the stick down. Dance with whatever's happening. It turns out, self-forgiveness will help you accept the things you cannot change.

Questions for Self-Discovery

- Which parenting styles do you relate to?
- What stories can you replace with up until now?
- What are signs you're getting triggered? How do you reclaim your brain?
- Are there ways you're still in denial?
- What's important about forgiveness in your story?
- How do you tend to beat yourself up?

CLAIRE'S STORY

Claire has always overcome any problem she encountered. She's the kind of person who takes on other people's challenges, and she always sees a path to success. When her child struggled, first in preschool and then in grade school, she hired an occupational therapist, started a social skills class, and established a mother-child group for third graders. Whenever a new problem was identified, she found a solution. Her child spent more time in medical offices than on the playground, but Claire was determined to do everything possible to help. By middle school, their relationship was strained, and by early high school, her child actively avoided and resisted her. As she pushed, things unraveled. Feeling defeated—she had tried everything!—she agreed to try parent training and coaching, and things started to improve quickly.

Bottom Line: Claire was determined to do everything in her power to help her child. But in her own words, "I thought I was getting help for my child. I didn't realize that the help was really for me."

CHAPTER 3

"I've Tried Everything, But Nothing Works"

Understanding and Redefining Parent Success

"But if we don't have the time and the willingness to take care of ourselves, how can we offer any genuine care to the people we love?" —THICH NHAT HANH

Relationships Are Suffering

We struggle to communicate well with the people we love the most—partners, kids, parents—precisely because they matter to us the most. We yell more than we'd like, avoid important conversations, cry when no one is around. The one thing we want most, to feel like our family functions as a team, is missing. Add to that a world of unmet expectations, difficulty in managing the daily logistics of family life, and fear for our children's future—it's no wonder our relationships can become a hot mess!

Relationships are challenging for complex kids *and* adults. They require time, patience, attention, intention, commitment, self-regulation, self-awareness, stamina, and other skills that depend on executive function (see Chapter 7). The very problems we're facing—executive dysfunction and emotional dysregulation—interfere with our ability to navigate relationship nuances.

Parents often come to Diane and me because the threads that connect family members to each other are fraying. They want to repair things before the connection breaks. They say

- "There is so much tension in our home."
- "Our marriage is struggling."
- "I just want her to talk to me."
- "He's out of control and it scares me."
- "I'm worried."
- "I'm at a loss."
- "I feel all alone."
- "She's in her own world and withdraws."
- "He won't eat with the family anymore."
- "I just want a happy family."
- "I just want a good relationship with my kid!"

Relationship challenges surface whether kids have a diagnosis or not. For children and teens with a clinical explanation for their challenges, it has usually been a long path to diagnosis. Parents have spent months or years seeking advice, searching for answers, and trying remedies, therapies, or good old-fashioned discipline to "fix" their child's unwanted behaviors. They are spent, and their patience has worn thin.

For children and teens who've never received an assessment, missed diagnosis often results in strained family relationships. Young people fumble into adulthood, stuck in a vortex of dependency and ineffective self-management. Parents may fear a danger in "labeling" their kids; others just don't know where to turn for guidance. Whatever the underlying cause, it's hard to address something if you don't know what it is.

Maybe we feel disconnected from ourselves or those we love. Maybe we feel ineffective as parents raising kids whose behaviors are surprising and uncomfortable. Maybe our kids feel out of control or worry they're a constant disappointment to us. The friction permeates all aspects of our relationships. It's extremely difficult to be the adults our kids need us to be. Here are some common ways this plays out:

- We hold on too tightly because we are desperate for our kids to be successful, robbing them of the opportunity to experience resilience without shame.
- We let go too soon because we think they need to learn how to take care of themselves, missing the chance to guide their development with encouragement.

- We focus on the tasks that need to get done at the expense of our connection, driving a wedge between us and our kids that's difficult to overcome.

Relationships in complex families may be taxed, but they're redeemable. You can reconnect with your kids and change your approach, so that you become the "good fit" your quirky kid needs. And you can communicate clearly and respectfully, authentically earning your child's respect. Because, what kids want most of all—at the heart of their relationships—is to feel respected and connected, starting at home.

Coach's Reframe: Change Starts with You

During the 2019 ADHD Parent's Palooza, Linda Roggli (ADDiva) and I had the privilege of interviewing leading researcher Dr. Stephen Hinshaw. I was riveted to his insights, especially as he spoke about a key notion from psychological research: "goodness of fit." Groundbreaking research in the 1950s and 1960s about temperament led to the understanding that it's important for parents and kids to "fit" together. "Goodness of fit" is essential to a child's emotional development.

"What really matters," explained Hinshaw, is "how much you mesh with and appreciate the temperament of your kid . . . It's not the parents or the kids *per se*. It's the blend. It's the fit." He continued, "The challenge for parenting any kid who's got some differences from other kids is appreciating your kid's difference, quirkiness, impulsivity, high activity level, [and] creativity." It's fundamental to building relationships that support kids who are different.

When kids don't meet typical developmental milestones (see Chapter 9), we usually want them to adapt, to fit with our approach to parenting. But research indicates that young people need us to adapt to fit them—their style, their proclivities, and their interests. When kids feel out of sync with their

> You have a unique, individual relationship with your child, no matter who else is involved.

parents, they can end up feeling like a "mis-fit" in their own family (pun intended.)

Do you ever offer help to your kids in a way that seems to push them away? As if no matter how hard you try, you can't seem to figure out what you can do to help? More than likely, it's not what you're doing, it's how. *How* we approach them and their challenges influences their willingness to accept our help.

I'm not saying that your reactions have caused your kids' challenges. But how you respond from here can set the tone for how your child learns to handle and overcome challenges moving forward. To change their behaviors, start by shifting your approach.

The parenting styles discussed in Chapter 2 are common, though not always helpful. But chances are, you also have moments of excellence and grace as a parent. Sometimes you respond calmly and confidently, instead of reacting. This book is designed to help you connect to (and cultivate) your inner conscious parent.

I invite you to expand into that part of yourself that's ready and able to parent from a place of clarity and consciousness. Meet Conscious Connie and Conscious Carl:

> **CONSCIOUS PARENT:** You're aware that life is chaotic, and that's okay. You're doing the best you can, and that's good enough, even though it's not perfect. You have immense gratitude, focusing on what's good in your life instead of what "could be." You have a "bring it on" attitude, tackling challenges with grace. You say, "This is my life, and there's so much that is good about it."

Think about your approach as a parent, your interactions with your kid, and how you typically respond to their challenges. You'll probably notice things you feel you're doing wrong, and that's okay. Now, what about things you're doing right? Can you identify your successes and your sweet spots? Give yourself credit for successes? Successes are where your best solutions are hidden (see Chapter 10), so focus on them to move things forward.

As you read this, it's possible you'll feel a little hopeless or worried because you and your coparent aren't on the same page. I get that. It's always worth working toward the goal of collaborative parenting. But I want to say this clearly: it only takes one parent to turn the ship. You have a unique, individual relationship with your child, no matter who else is involved. You can create a strong relationship that supports your child, even if your coparent is not (yet) on board. The bottom line to effective parenting is simple: change starts with you.

For the rest of this book, think about your goals and your approach without judging yourself for anything you've done up until now. Focus on understanding your role, on the changes you want to create. Search for a new path

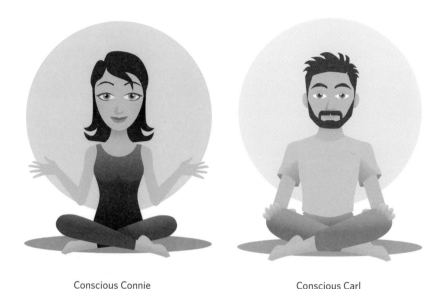

Conscious Connie   Conscious Carl

to grow into the kind of parent your kids need, which is ultimately the kind of parent you want to be.

Raising complex kids is an unexpected life adventure. It's going to require some course correction. Who better than you to lead the way?

Strategy: Relationships over Tasks

Walking through our family room while my three kids were sitting on the couch watching television, I was annoyed they were sitting there laughing when I had so much to do. Honestly, there was nothing they really needed to do at that time, and there was no reason for me to engage. But I did. I started looking around for something for them to do.

They were (rightfully) annoyed when I directed them to shut off the TV and then ordered them around the house. They let me know in no uncertain terms as they begrudgingly slammed down the remote and moved to action.

In hindsight, my need for them to be "busy" or "productive" was my problem, not theirs. I honestly can't remember what chores or homework I insisted on, but I'm certain it really didn't have to be done that exact moment. I didn't have to interrupt them or step on their fun. In that moment, I made unloading the dishwasher or doing homework more important than my relationship with them.

What does allowing them to watch television have to do with our relationship? I was making tasks—getting stuff done—more important than their interests, needs, self-esteem, and autonomy, for no real reason other than to calm my own anxiety.

Focusing too much on tasks can cause damage to our relationships with our kids, spouses, and coparents. We get so caught up in the business of our lives, with what we think is right, that we forget they're independent human beings on their own paths, with their own perspectives and desires. When we hyperfocus on tasks (even tasks that are important), we lose site of the bigger picture—staying connected.

For example:

- We fuss at a teen for leaving a wet towel on the floor *again* in a tone that communicates "you're lazy."
- We force a late night to finish homework, long after a child is clearly beyond capacity, sending a message that communicates "try harder."
- We send kids to go get socks, and then greet them with a message that communicates "why can't you just get it together?" when they come back empty handed (or worse, with a toy in hand).

Sure we want to teach kids to pick up wet towels, have them complete their homework, and put strategies in place to support their working memory. But we're more likely to help them learn these skills when our relationships are strong and we're working together collaboratively.

Throughout dozens of interviews with thought leaders in the fields of ADHD and parenting during the 2019 ADHD Parent's Palooza, Drs. Ned Hallowell, Stephen Hinshaw, Roberto Olivardia, Carolyn Parcells, and others struck a consistent theme: stay connected. There's almost nothing more important that parents can do, they said, than focus on their relationships with their complex kids.

Relationships are built on trust, which releases oxytocin, a "happy hormone" that makes kids available to learning, research shows. Discord and disharmony release cortisol, a "stress hormone" that interferes with trust and learning.

The secret to parenting complex kids—any kids, really—is to lean into the relationship. That doesn't mean "be their best friend," "give them everything they want," or "don't teach them to be responsible." It means maintaining respectful, open, healthy communication. Strong relationships tell our kids that we have their backs. When our children trust us, they know we're doing our best for them and that we won't lead them down a path that's not in their best interest. They can choose to trust us, even when they don't agree with us.

A trusting relationship tells our kids it's okay to be themselves, to mess up, to try, to fail, to succeed—because we will be there with our love unconditionally, even when they don't get all the tasks done!

Say No to Defensiveness (Don't Take the Bait)

Years ago, my husband and I were out of sync, both stuck in defense mode. I have no idea who "started it," but our conversations were limited to logistics. Our shields were up, and our connection was down. I was aware of the distance between us, but it felt safer to stay hidden behind sandbags than to risk the rising flood.

This probably sounds familiar. Many of us live in a chronic state of defense. In fact, we constantly use military references in our daily human interactions: *lower your shields, pick your battles, call a truce, stick to your guns, take the first shot, send in the reinforcements, détentes*—not to mention *battle of the sexes*! But these analogies create a zero-sum gain in relationships; rather than victory, they lock us in unending conflict.

Do you really *want* to be "doing battle" with your teenager or 10-year-old, spouse or parent, supervisor or employee?

Relationships flourish when we remove roadblocks. It's time to pull your important relationships out of the barracks. Start with an olive branch, but be patient. When we get locked in a crisply starched uniform, we forget how to stand at ease. Even as you start to treat your loved ones as allies, it can take some time for them to step off the battlefield.

> One of the greatest superpowers you can cultivate is to *stop taking things personally.*

Thankfully, my spouse saw the signs and began looking for common ground. He talked and smiled more. Because my shields were well established, it took time for me to lay down my sword and stop taking things personally. He waited without re-arming himself; instead, he met me with virtual flowers and a box of chocolates. Eventually my shields came down and our connection improved. But it took a while.

COACH YOURSELF TO STOP TAKING THE BAIT

One of the greatest superpowers you can cultivate is to *stop taking things personally*. I took everything (yes, everything) personally when my kids were little, and it was exhausting. But when I finally accepted that "other people's stuff is their stuff," and it's not about me, it was positively liberating.

When a family member or student pushes your buttons, usually they're not doing it manipulatively (even if you think they are). When you "take the bait," they get the results they want, a distraction from whatever was making them uncomfortable. It's up to you to resist the temptation to let it become about you. They may be pushing, but the buttons are yours.

A fundamental component of the coach approach is simply this: keep yourself out of it. As Wendy Mogel says in *The Blessing of a Skinned Knee*, whenever possible we want to "remain calm, casual, firm and matter-of-fact."

Say Yes to Redefining Success

"Success is liking yourself, liking what you do, and liking how you do it."
—Maya Angelou

In the early years of the twenty-first century, Dr. David Rock wrote in *Psychology Today*, "People everywhere seem to be experiencing an epidemic of overwhelm." He pointed to two explanations: the volume of information we process and the cost of distractions. And that was written *before* every child had a supercomputer in their pocket.

We process something like 70,000 thoughts per day, and we are exposed to excessive amounts of new information in an interruption-driven environment of social media and technology. Consider how that impacts people with complex brains and lagging executive function skills! And yet, somehow, we continue to hold Ozzie and Harriet as the gold standard in a world moving at the speed of George and Jane Jetson.

We're moving fast as lightning, trying to respond to the stimuli coming at us. But breakneck speed is an unsustainable course. It's not that I don't want success. It's just that, to be honest, life in the twenty-first century, even with all of our time-saving technologies, feels like we're constantly playing dodgeball while being expected to serve the perfect game of tennis on the same court.

Today's performance expectations fly in the face of reason. It's unreasonable to expect ourselves to achieve mastery in nearly every aspect of our lives. And yet we do. This is all the more unfair for our complex kids, who are often specialists living in a generalists' world.

HOW TO *NOT* TAKE THINGS PERSONALLY

When you notice yourself taking things personally, use these questions and suggestions as a guide. For example, if you ask your son to fold the laundry and he responds, "I'll do it later":

What's the message you're telling yourself? "He's irresponsible," or "he'll never do it," or "yeah, right!" If you feel like you're not being a good parent if he doesn't do it now, you'll feel compelled to nag to make sure he gets it done. What are you really worried about?

What else is also true about this situation? It might also be true that he intends to do it, but he forgets. Or that he didn't process what you said because you didn't have his attention. Or that he is embarrassed that he's not good at folding clothes. Get curious.

Respond supportively instead of defensively. Instead of snide comments, acknowledge, "That's great. Thank you. When will you have it done?" If he's evasive ("I don't know, Mom, just later!"), then help establish the time frame matter-of-factly ("I'd really like it done by X time—does that sound reasonable?"). Give him as much control as possible.

Show you're on his team and you want to help. Instead of feeling slighted or disrespected, ask your child, "Is there any help you need from me? Would you like a reminder?" He may resist your attempts at first, so keep your focus on matter-of-fact, positive communication. If he resists, give him a little time and ask again, this time acknowledging that he's probably frustrated, and remind him you're trying to help without nagging.

My life is no different from yours. We're all feeling it: the realm of unreasonable expectations. It's almost as if we are setting ourselves up for failure, but then we're shocked to discover it's a possible outcome.

What does it look like to redefine success in this era?

- Let things go.
- Get clear on what's really important.
- Embrace "good enough" when appropriate (see Chapter 8).
- Say no to constant obligations.
- Loosen up when things just don't matter.
- Choose where to focus instead of trying to focus on everything.

Ultimately, redefining success means setting our own expectations instead of looking to the outside world to define them for us. It means basing those expectations on our values or passions rather than on some prescribed societal norms that tell us what we're supposed to do.

When I talk with groups of parents about success, there's general agreement that we would all benefit from lightening the load on our kids and on ourselves as parents. So the time has come to renegotiate our relationship with perfectionism, reacquaint ourselves with new ideals of excellence, and redefine what success looks like in this modern world. For example, putting time limits on homework can prevent twelve-year-olds from burning the midnight oil; celebrating a child's efforts can reduce the sting of a test that doesn't go so well.

Success is in the mind of the beholder. I challenge you to redefine it in terms of what is beneficial for your kids. Let go of your own (and others') preconceived notions and begin creating new expectations that come from knowing your kids for who they are, rather than someone else's "shoulds."

As a recovering perfectionist, this is hard for me (see Chapter 8). Every day I make the effort to redefine success in terms that make sense for my family, and for me.

- I remind my husband that a 90 is still an A when he judges his own performance too harshly.
- I encourage my dyslexic daughter to be thrilled with a B on a Lit paper.
- And I own my mistakes vocally and make the effort to forgive myself ... daily.

That's what I call success.

Self-Talk: Trust Your Instincts

I got off to a rocky start with parenting, starting in pregnancy and continuing for more than a decade. To say I wasn't a confident parent is a vast understatement. I worried about everything. I didn't trust that my kids were getting enough food or growing appropriately. I questioned whether I was doing *anything* right at all. Whatever confidence I might have mustered going into parenting was gone by the time my first child was six months old.

I spent the first 10 years dancing with doubt, governed by an internal script: "What if they find out that you have no idea what you're doing? What if you're messing up these kids and it's all your fault that they're having such a hard time?"

The person whose opinion I needed to trust the most was the one I trusted the least—me.

Occasionally I'd have good days or weeks, but inevitably something would happen with one of my kiddos that would derail me and throw me back into the depths of self-doubt. My definition of success was a perfectionist ideal, and my sense of self-worth was inextricably linked with it: when my kids were hitting appropriate milestones, I was a good mom. When they were failing to hit milestones, I was a bad mom.

Truly my sense of myself was only as strong as any one of my children's worst day.

Our lives have changed dramatically in the dozen-plus years since I discovered that believing in myself and trusting myself was the secret ingredient to effective parenting. Truth is, I had to learn to trust myself as a parent. It didn't come naturally.

Learning to trust your instincts is an essential part of the coach approach, a way of parenting that works for you and your kids. You may not feel it at first, but it's okay to "fake it 'til you make it." Because as you begin to lead yourself, you'll begin to lead your family with confidence.

What is it to trust your instincts?

- Allow yourself to make decisions and take action based on your own values or compass.
- Live according to your own expectations, not everyone else's.
- Know that whatever comes up, you are resourceful enough to figure out how to handle it.

- Let go of needing to know what's going to happen, and trust you'll make clear decisions when needed.

How do you actually trust your own instincts?

- Set clear, consistent expectations and communicate them; be flexible enough to roll with changes as they arise. Inevitably they will.
- Apologize and take responsibility for your mistakes. You don't need to exert control when you're operating from internal authority.
- Let go of your need to be right and for your kids to be perfect. Teach your kids to learn from mistakes without blame or shame.

Kids do best when their parents believe things are going to be okay. When kids see their parents acting with confidence (rather than controlling out of fear), it fosters cooperation and trust, inviting them to believe in themselves.

If you have stepped (even occasionally) into confidence and learned to trust your instincts when raising complex kids, *please* take a moment to celebrate. Give yourself some credit. It's not easy to do when you get so many messages to the contrary.

If you're not feeling confident, if you're worried about your child's self-esteem, if you're second-guessing your decisions, or if you're never quite comfortable with the choices you're making, I want to invite you to get some help to do something different. Start with one step. Attend a retreat, join a coaching group, register for online parent training, start morning affirmations, read the blog on ImpactParents.com, commit to finishing this book—do something to help you build your confidence, one step at a time.

I speak from experience: confidence is a muscle you can strengthen. When you do, everyone in your family will benefit.

Questions for Self-Discovery

- Which of your relationships would you like to improve?
- What does "change starts with you" mean to you?
- How do tasks interfere with your relationships?
- When do you tend to take things personally?
- How do you want to redefine success?
- When do you trust your instincts?

MARC AND GWEN'S STORY

Marc and Gwen are accomplished, high-achieving, ambitious professionals, and they expected their children to follow suit. Their oldest, a high-achieving athlete, is a straight-A student, albeit a bit high strung. Their youngest, however, is a stereotypical 11-year-old boy with ADHD. He's distracted, impulsive, messy, and still unconcerned with doing well in school. He doesn't care much about athletics, though his father pushes him to compete. Getting his sister triggered is easy and arguably his favorite sport, though his parents don't see her responses as overreactions. As Marc and Gwen continuously interrupt and correct each other, it's clear that they agree on one thing: their son is the only person in the entire family with a "problem."

Bottom Line: Their youngest child is an 11-year-old boy with ADHD. "If he would just . . . " is their most common refrain.

CHAPTER 4

"I Just Want Some Peace!"

The Four Phases of Parenting

"Looking without judgment, we can understand, and compassion is born." —THICH NHAT HANH

The Experts Don't Live in Your House

One rainy night in 2005, I attended a talk by my favorite parenting author, Wendy Mogel, author of *The Blessing of a Skinned Knee*. As she spoke about building resilience and letting kids "fail," I raised my hand with tears in my eyes. "What if your child has special needs?" I asked. She replied, "Then this doesn't apply to you."

I was stunned. I don't know what else was said that night. The tears kept coming. "If this doesn't apply to me," I thought, "what does?"

I had ventured into the world of parenting with sepia-tinted images of laughing at the antics of my small children and rose-tinted visions of my teens requesting words of wisdom from their cool mom. My life was going to be a Kodak commercial.

Was I overly optimistic or ridiculously naïve? I think I was pretty typical.

I was caught off guard when the challenges started. I read books, consulted experts, and tried to follow traditional parenting advice with each new problem as it arose. But as I've heard echoed from countless clients over the years, traditional parenting advice doesn't always work for nontraditional kids. In fact, sometimes it backfires. My client captured it clearly: "He had been such a happy, outgoing kid. But when he got angry in response to our setting limits, the doctor told us to set more limits. We did, and things just kept getting worse and worse. I can honestly say I felt like the worst parent in the world."

I, too, felt like a failure as a parent. When traditional parenting guidance didn't improve things, I began to lose hope. I feared for my child's future, worried about everything. Would my child:

- be able to manage life independently?
- make it through school, through college, and into a career?
- maintain relationships and raise a family?
- do something impulsive (read: dangerous) that would ruin prospects for a happy life?
- end up living in my basement for the rest of their life?

I did receive some very helpful support and expertise. I was relieved when I found professionals who had lived the life and "got it." Other times, even the most well-meaning professionals didn't provide the guidance I needed—not because they didn't care or weren't well informed, but because complex kids are complicated. I needed more than just treatment for symptoms. I needed big-picture help to learn how to develop workable solutions.

My kids needed me to understand that they weren't being "naughty" (see Chapter 6), they were struggling. I wanted their teachers, coaches, babysitters, doctors, friends' parents, and family members to understand that too.

Everything changed as I gradually grew to understand that for complex kids:

- Positive parenting is not enough (though it's essential).
- Adults need to set realistic expectations.
- Solutions are best when individualized.
- Systems need flexibility without compromising accountability.

The experts are going to tell you what they think you should do, but they don't actually know what's going on in your house at 6:00 pm. You do. So, gather information, think it through, and explore your options. And then remember, information isn't enough to create lasting change. What you really want is transformation.

Traditional parenting gurus offer amazing advice. I owe so much to the wisdom of thought leaders such as Wendy Mogel and Hal Runkel. Still, whenever you listen to the wisdom of the sages of parenting (including the ideas found in this book), make sure it makes sense for your kid!

Mogel's talk helped me understand it was time to stop trying to fit my kids into a traditional parenting mold. They didn't fit. Instead I had to create a new mold that worked for them and me.

Coach's Reframe: Parent Like a Coach

In an effort to support parents struggling with complex kids, in my 40s I started coach training with the Co-Active Training Institute (CTI). Within hours, I was hooked; within weeks, communication with my family improved dramatically. Just over a dozen years later, in a 2019 interview in *Flaunt Magazine*, my eldest brought me to tears with their appreciation for what coaching gave them:

> "Well, my parents are both life coaches. It started when I was about 12, and it's been beautiful to watch them evolve, and watch them grow and learn. Coaching has changed our entire family. Once they became coaches, all their time was dedicated to telling people, 'Follow your dreams, do what you need to do, do what's right for you, and take care of yourself.' They couldn't exactly tell me something different, and, fortunately, they realized that. So, all the work that they were doing with other people, they extended to me."

I realized that other parents needed to learn what we'd learned: Expert advice doesn't always work, but trusting ourselves generally does.

You know your child better than anyone. Truly you do. Your challenges are to learn to trust your instincts; listen to your child and to your heart; and, when necessary, ignore the experts and be the parent your child needs you to be.

Learning to parent in a way that worked for my family, I unearthed a transformational paradigm—the coach approach—that offers an effective way to manage difficult behaviors. It doesn't solve people's problems; it teaches them a foolproof method for problem solving. It has and will continue to change the landscape for parenting complex kids across the world.

A COACH APPROACH

Coaching is an evidence-based method for change management, helping people realize their full potential. For parents and educators, a coach approach applies the basic concepts, ideas, and strategies from coaching to support kids on their path to become independent, self-directed, and self-motivated adults. Four cornerstone concepts from coaching adapt beautifully when applied specifically to complex kids:

1. People aren't broken; they're creative, resourceful, and whole.
2. To create change, people must have ownership of their agenda.
3. Life's curveballs are to be expected and are an opportunity for growth and learning.
4. To address problems, we must look at how they relate to all aspects of our lives.

There's really nothing more you could want for your kids than to have them reach their full potential. You want them to understand what makes them tick without getting defensive; to believe in themselves; and to feel capable of becoming successful adults. As you learn to provide honest and constructive feedback in a way that kids can receive it, you'll communicate with less judgment and more acceptance. Kids will see you as a member of their team, and seek your guidance and support.

You can learn to:

- let go of fear and judgement;
- see your kids' capabilities and gifts;
- advocate for them effectively;
- set appropriate expectations and priorities;
- improve your communication;
- offer guidance your kids can accept without defensiveness;
- put systems into place that work well for everyone; and
- make it okay for them to make mistakes.

Your kids can learn to:

- take ownership of their lives with self-management skills;
- embrace their strengths and talents;
- find the motivation to focus on learning in school and life;
- overcome obstacles, set goals, and reach for them;
- improve relationships with family and peers; and
- become accountable, independent, and responsible.

A coach approach guides you to become the parent you want to be, and it helps you create the kind of relationship with your child that you've always wanted. You don't have to become a coach to do this. As you begin to adopt these principles and tools, a coach approach will enhance the rest of your life in stunning ways.

Strategy: The Four Phases of Parenting

Parenting doesn't happen in a straight line. Instead, parents move in and out of four key phases in relationship with their kids, gradually transferring ownership to them. But it's a complicated dynamic. Holding on too tightly is counterproductive to the goal of independence; providing the right amount of scaffolding without enabling or fostering a learned helplessness is an art.

> Effective parenting is not about controlling kids; it's about teaching them to take control of themselves.

Effective parenting is not about controlling kids; it's about teaching them to take control of themselves. Ideally, parents will consciously prepare children for independence so that their kids gradually take on the mantle of responsibility for themselves. Understanding the four phases guides parents in this process.

EMPOWERING INDEPENDENCE STEP BY STEP

Phase 1: Motivate effort and direct work. Parents hold the agenda for what's expected of the child, direct the child's actions and behaviors, and provide motivation for encouragement. All parents start off here, directing actions and behaviors to keep kids safe. Kids expect parents to be in charge. Parents may get stuck here because it's familiar, it's easy, or they worry things won't get done without them. As your child becomes capable of doing more for themselves, look for opportunities to move to the next phase.

Language directs action. *"Tonight you have math and spelling homework. Let's have a snack and do homework before dinner so we can play a game later."*

Phase 2: Motivate ownership and model organization. Collaborative efforts start with parents taking the lead and beginning to share the agenda with their child. Parents help kids find motivation to take some ownership and participate in planning. They cultivate independence, guide kids through problem-solving and decision-making activities, transfer ownership incrementally, and allow kids to experience increasing amounts of self-management. When you aren't sure what your kids need from you, phase 2 is a strong place to start.

> Language shifts from "we" to "you," adding open-ended questions. *"You can do your homework before or after dinner tonight. Do you know what you've got, or when you want to do it? Where? How will you reward yourself when you're done?"*

Phase 3: Transfer ownership and support organization. Collaboration continues. As kids take ownership of their agenda and practice self-management, parents practice letting go, moving into a support role. Teens often demand independence when they're ready for you to be in this phase. As the stakes get higher (such as with driving and college applications), parents are tempted to tighten the reins. Instead, ask permission to make suggestions and offer advice, empowering your teen's ownership and self-determination.

> Language makes it clear the child is in charge with a parent offering support. *"It looks like you're pretty much on top of things. How are you feeling? What's your plan for . . . ? Is there anything I can do to help?"* or *"I had a thought. Would you like to hear it?"*

Phase 4: Empower, champion, and troubleshoot. The teen or young adult is predominantly in control of their agenda, living an independent life, while parents encourage and offer problem-solving support as needed. There's a general understanding that parents are no longer responsible for routine management. Parents may begin to move into adult relationships with their kids in many arenas starting in the teen years, though it's not usually a reasonable expectation to fully move into this phase until a young adult's brain development is completed, around age 25 at the youngest.

> Language shifts to checking in and championing. *"How's it going? Looks like you're rocking things out these days. What are you celebrating this week? Anything I can help you with?"* or *"It looks like things are*

going well, but if you ever want to talk through anything, just know that I'm here."

Parents move in and out of the four phases, depending on their child's needs in specific circumstances. As examples:

- You're feeling like a drill sergeant in the mornings (phase 1). You think your 7-year-old is ready for more independence, so together you agree to start working on getting dressed independently and strategize to help them do that (phase 2).
- Your 11-year-old still needs your help getting started on their math homework (phase 2), but they are motivated by soccer and get ready without reminders (phase 3).
- Your 16-year-old is handling junior year independently (phase 3), but during exams you sense they're struggling and hesitant to ask for support. You suggest a planning session to help them get back on track (phase 2).
- If your kid is demanding independence but you find yourself wondering, "is it okay to let my child fail?" spend a little time collaboratively planning (phase 2) before you shift roles and let them take the lead (phase 3).
- If you have been successfully hands-off (phase 3) and notice your child start to struggle, don't jump in and take over (phase 1). Instead downshift to collaboratively ask questions and guide them (phase 2). Move back into a support role gradually, in small steps (phase 3).
- Even independent college kids (phase 4) may need your help in stressful times. During sophomore year, my daughter called in a panic. I didn't tell her what to do (phase 1) or what I could do to help (phase 2). I asked, "What support is available to you right now?" (phase 3). She decided to make an appointment with Student Support, and I checked in later to confirm she was back on track (phase 4).

As we adapt *our* behaviors according to these four phases, we transfer ownership and encourage kids to take on new levels of independence. Read the signs and meet your kids where they are, providing the appropriate collaboration and support to allow them the most independence they're able to handle.

Say No to Judgment

Dr. Ned Hallowell refers to stigmatizing the behaviors of complex kids as a "moral diagnosis"—the tendency to judge kids' behaviors as wrong, when in fact they're behaviors that kids have not yet learned to control. Such judgments are passed by strangers, family members, teachers, and sometimes even parents, causing lasting emotional scars. And when we don't give kids an explanation for their challenges and their behaviors, they'll judge themselves, too, usually with something much uglier than the truth.

As adults, we do this to ourselves, as well. We judge ourselves harshly, showing equal disdain for both little and major mistakes.

Judgment is a challenging concept, full of contradictions.

- We use judgment to guide us in our lives every day. We categorize our experiences into good, bad, and neutral, and that leads us to certain behaviors and decisions. In many ways, it makes life easier.
- As Dr. Mark Bertin explains in his book, *The ADHD Family Solution*, judgment "leads us to wrestle with what is not in our control." For example, it's understandable that parents of children with challenges feel disappointed when they can't control their children's behaviors. If a hyperactive 10-year-old is bouncing off the walls or jumping on the furniture, frustrated parents may come to the judgment that this kid is disrespectful and won't listen to them; or worse, that he'll never live up to his potential.

"Standing in judgment" does not serve our children—or us. Attaching a stigma to a behavior makes them feel like a failure, interfering with our ability to help them learn to improve that behavior.

The judgment we feel for our children is also painful and disheartening for us as parents. As we lose hope and confidence in their future, we become disappointed and question ourselves as parents. We fear we must be doing something wrong or things would be better for our kids. We conflate their success with our own.

So, what's a parent to do? How do you redirect your child's behaviors and foster resilience and self-confidence at the same time? What if you were to fully accept that recognizing and supporting your kids in their struggles is actually the mark of good parenting?

Dr. Bertin encourages parents to replace judgment with discernment. "Discernment is recognizing what we can and should change, and what we cannot, much like the traditional serenity prayer: To accept what we cannot change, to change what we must, and to find the wisdom to tell the difference."

For parents, that means fully understanding our child's challenges and accepting them for what they are. And it means helping our children learn self-management, slowly but surely, in developmentally appropriate ways, one step at a time. We'll talk about this in many ways throughout the book, especially in Chapter 6.

Although there is no magic wand for stepping out of judgment, it helps to pay attention to your tone and to underlying messages you may be unintentionally sending. When you stop your hyperactive child from trying to see if he can fit in the laundry chute, examine your thoughts and feelings at that time. Are you aggravated? Annoyed? Or are you laughing at your child's insatiable curiosity and incredible energy? Your thoughts—and the words and tones that follow them—communicate volumes.

Say Yes to Different Perspectives

"The truth of most truths is that they are perception and not, in fact, true."
—Simon Sinek

Have you ever experienced one of those classic moments in the grocery store when your child is melting down and everyone is staring at you? Judging you and your screaming kid? What goes through your mind? Is your gut instinct to judge your child as well? Or yourself? Can your child see the judgment on your face or hear it in your voice?

In that moment, what's your perspective? Are you thinking about how people might be judging you? Fair enough. It's embarrassing, to say the least.

You could also think to yourself, "This kid is having a really hard time. How can I help them manage these intense emotions?" That perspective may not stop others from staring, but it could help you get through the situation in a positive way that strengthens your relationship with your child.

When we look at things from different perspectives, it opens up the possibility for new outcomes. You've probably heard the expression, "perspectives influence reality." In actuality, perspectives have the capacity to change reality.

You have a choice. Every moment of every day, you are making choices, even when you think you have no choice. For example, you don't really *have to* do the dishes every day. You may choose to have a clean kitchen because you like the way it feels, but that's actually a choice.

It's freeing to recognize your choices and begin to take ownership of them. Besides, it's almost impossible to make sustainable change in your life without changing your underlying thoughts or perspective. As Henry Ford stated, "whether you believe you can, or believe you can't, you're right."

> Every moment of every day, you are making choices, even when you think you have no choice.

For example, if you think "my son is disrespectful because he never does what I ask him to do," then you're going to approach him as if he's disrespectful. But if you change that perspective and consider a new thought, such as "my son doesn't do what I say because he struggles with memory issues, and then he gets rude because he's embarrassed that he forgot," you might approach things differently.

If you think your child *can* do something, or if you think *you can* stop yelling, it's amazing how much more easily that becomes a reality. But if you think you can't—or they can't—well, you get the idea. To create a new perspective, you have to believe that it could be true. If you really don't believe your son is struggling or embarrassed, then you're not really taking on that perspective.

Here's the best part: You have complete control over your perspective and can change it at any time—with a little conscious effort, of course.

In fact, I'm modeling it throughout this book. In each chapter, I present a "problem" that's familiar to most of us. And then I offer a "coach's reframe," another way of looking at that problem. Reframing the problem is a way of considering a different perspective, encouraging us to explore new possibilities. We won't necessarily stop seeing the problems that we face, but if we look at them through different lenses, we'll begin to see opportunities emerge alongside them.

Sometimes we get stuck in perspectives that we don't even realize we're taking. When you notice that you're attached to a perspective, ask yourself "how else can I look at this?" or "what else is also true?" Notice what happens. When you shift perspectives, you change what's possible, and that will lead to different results.

Self-Talk: Letting Go

For their senior year of high school, my oldest child, who has significant executive function challenges, attended a 2E (Twice Exceptional) school in Los Angeles, CA, and lived with a family in order to pursue acting. I lived in Atlanta, Georgia.

In January, they got a job that required relocation to a city in another country for several months. It was an incredible opportunity for them professionally—a dream come true. But they had never worked, lived alone, done school independently, or been responsible for feeding themselves. It was all I could do not to panic.

I chose to see it as a tremendous opportunity for them to rise to the occasion. Their motivation was strong, so we collaborated to help them achieve success.

We talked about what they could handle independently. Bex was confident they could make it to work on time (even though getting to school had been a problem), so we talked about how they'd achieve success in that area and agreed that I'd check in occasionally. They were confident they could learn their lines on their own and make sure to get enough sleep, so I stepped out of that completely.

Bex felt three things were too much to manage independently: getting meals when not on set, finances, and doing schoolwork. I agreed to help as much as possible. We came up with a plan that involved a lot of microwave meals (not easy for a strictly gluten-free person in 2013); we figured out the finances and how they would share information; and I got to work finding a tutor. The arrangement comforted both of us. I had Bex's permission to be involved, and Bex knew I had their back. I focused on those things Bex asked me to handle, which enabled me to let go of other things with slightly more confidence and ease.

Parenting is a daily exercise in letting go: letting go of control, letting go of unrealistic expectations, letting go of kids doing things the way we think they should, and letting go of how we appear to others.

It's like transferring batons in the long relay race of childhood. We start off holding all the batons, responsible for everything. Then we transfer batons, one by one, to their rightful owners—our kids. We want to make sure kids grasp each baton firmly, so don't throw it (even when you're tempted). You want to pass it carefully so your kids can take hold with confidence.

THE ART OF LETTING GO

These four questions can guide you to finding a comfort zone with transferring ownership. You're not always going to like it, but clear expectations make it manageable. With every step your child takes toward independence, recalibrate your response to match their changing world.

Where Can I Let Go Next? What's the next issue for your child to take on? Choose one place to transfer ownership. What would independence look like? How will you know they've achieved it? It's tempting to expect kids to take on everything at once, so focus on pacing yourself. (See Chapter 5.)

Where Do I Want to Continue Holding On? Collaborate with your kids to clarify which batons they still need you to hold and where they might need scaffolding. Identify what they're ready for that you might still be holding onto.

How Can I Help? Turn to your child for guidance. Ask them what they want from you in terms of support. At first they may not know, but asking will help them think about what they need, empowering them to learn to use support when appropriate. If they resist support, ask yourself question 2 again. Are they ready for more than you're giving them?

What Do I Need to Feel Comfortable? Letting go of the need to be in control is harder for some of us than others, so take care of yourself. Get support or coaching for yourself. Look for what will give you comfort in the process, because when you're feeling anxious or uptight, you're likely to hold on too tight, for too long.

When you are too attached to your kids' success, you risk holding on too tight or too long. You must be willing to give up a little control so you can transfer ownership to your kids. That's our job as parents. But it's not easy. Most of us have worked hard to gain a sense of control in our lives, so letting go may cause internal conflict.

Questions for Self-Discovery

- How are you an expert for your family?
- What's the benefit of parenting like a coach?
- Which parenting phase are you in generally? Which phase is your child ready for you to move into?
- How does judgment inadvertently show up in your parenting?
- What perspectives keep you stuck?
- What or when do you want to let go?

PART 2

The Impact Model

A NEW PARADIGM FOR PARENTING LIKE A COACH

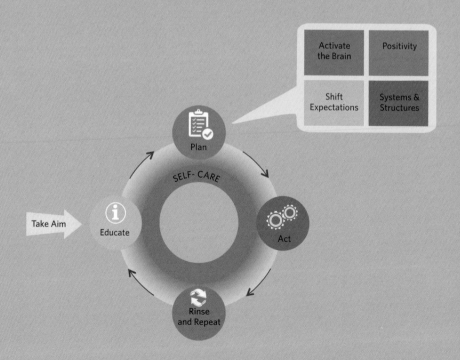

How to Tackle Challenging Situations

At the core of the coach approach is the six-step Impact Model. It offers a clear, simple structure to address challenging situations—one success at a time.

Step 1: Take AIM. Focus on one challenge at a time, the more specific the better. Ask yourself, "What's the change I want to see?"

Step 2: Get Educated. Collect information to understand the context around a problem. Prepare for problem-solving by exploring perspectives from you, your child, and others.

Step 3: Plan. Every challenge could have multiple solutions. Explore these cornerstones before taking action:

Activate the Brain: Kids' brains influence all of their thoughts and behaviors (also true for stressed-out adults). Ask yourself, "What role is their brain playing?" and "How can we support or activate their complex brain?"

Positivity: With constant redirection and correction, relationships with kids are taxed. Envision their potential. Empower them to believe in their own success. Ask yourself, "What are their strengths?" and "What successes can we celebrate?"

Shift Expectations: When kids are developmentally delayed, set high expectations appropriately and incrementally. Ask yourself, "Is that a realistic expectation based on the child's developmental age?"

Systems and Structures: Use systems and structures in the context of activating the brain, positivity, and shifting expectations, to help kids learn self-management and self-regulation. Ask yourself, "What's the goal of creating a new system?"

Step 4: Act. Get started, taking action on the plan!

Step 5: Rinse and Repeat. Real and lasting change takes practice, time, and experimentation. Try something, tweak it, and try again. When you're ready, take aim on something new.

Step 6: Self Care. Taking care of yourself is essential for your stamina and resilience, and to model conscious self-management for kids.

JENNA'S STORY

Jenna was struggling to manage her reactions. Her 14-year-old twins were becoming increasingly disrespectful, and she knew that yelling and threatening weren't helpful. Then she had a magical moment. On a group coaching call, she explained, "It was as if I could hear the lightbulb going off in my head. I thought, 'use the model.' And then I laughed out loud, channeled Elaine's voice, and asked myself, 'what's the change I want to see?'" Jenna decided to Take Aim on helping her kids respond respectfully when they heard "no," especially when she was asking them to do something they wouldn't want to do. She got curious about the source of her kids' snarky behaviors and acknowledged how often she was taking things personally. She and her kids agreed on a code word to prepare for disappointment, and she was already noticing improvement. "Once I remembered to use the model, everything started to get better quickly," she said. She was beginning to coach herself.

Bottom Line: "I thought, 'use the model.'" And then, clearly and quietly, she asked herself, "What's the change I want to see?"

CHAPTER 5

"Where Do I Start?"

You Can Do It All, but Not at the Same Time (Take Aim)

> "We are often completely focused on preventing the event we dread,
> and we forget that joy is also possible even in an
> unpredictable world." —THICH NHAT HANH

The Sheer Volume Is Daunting

The early years of parenting were completely overwhelming for me. Routine requirements to keep a household running smoothly were extensive (and not unique to me): school and homework, sports and cultural activities, playdates, meal planning, laundry, carpooling, working, religious education, extended family, supporting each other, basic health care, paying the bills, being a good neighbor and friend, clothes shopping, food shopping, and more.

Raising children taxes any parent's capacity for organization, self-management, and overall emotional management!

When you add a family member with complex challenges into the mix, it stretches the limits even further. And when an adult has their own challenges, too, they often bulge at the seams with the added weight of responsibility (see Chapter 2).

Basic parenting is magnified when kids are:

- bouncing off the furniture and the walls;
- losing everything from lunch boxes to coats to socks (oh, the socks!);
- having epic meltdowns long past their toddler years;
- clinging tightly to their parents, hesitant to face the world independently; and/or

- annoying parents and teachers by staring off into space, jumping too quickly into action, or reacting so intensely the family feels they're walking on eggshells.

In addition to the fundamentals of family life, complex kids come with a host of other responsibilities required of parents:

- support for school challenges;
- additional teacher and school meetings;
- advocating for school accommodations;
- additional medical appointments, assessments, therapies, and tutors;
- supervising playdates;
- responding to meltdowns and upsets;
- explaining kids to extended family members, coaches, and teachers;
- family arguments and upsets;
- extra emotional support;
- staying while kids fall asleep;
- helping kids manage even the most basic routines;
- setting up routines that work for specific kids; and
- parent training, coaching, and support.

Simply put, kids who are wired to be impulsive, clingy, distracted, disorganized, fearful, emotionally unregulated, and/or hyperactive can wreak havoc in the life of a family, requiring a great deal more than typical parenting.

And those are just the things parents are responsible for. It doesn't include all the things that kids need to learn to do for themselves (that parents need to teach them). That's where the real challenge comes in for many parents—how to help kids in a way that they'll receive it.

Beyond the extra burden of supporting and advocating for special needs, there is an emotional load on parents of complex kids that is difficult to articulate, and it carries the heaviest weight of all—worry.

Usually, parents have had a sense that "something is not quite right" for quite some time. They are scared, angry, overwhelmed, or all three. They are ready (read: desperate) for something to change. And they want it to change now, before it's too late!

Many parents feel an urgency to address all of their kids' issues at once. Concern that their kids won't be ready for the future compels them to double-down on action (or discipline). So they apply pressure, to themselves and their kids, which compounds the problems. Trying to tackle everything at once seems like the only solution; and yet it makes things worse, not better.

The simple truth is this: when there are complex issues in the house, the struggle is real!

Coach's Reframe: Take a Marathon View

Anyone who has participated in a long-distance event—and I must admit that does not include me—will tell you that you don't just show up on the day of the event. And when you pace yourself in a race, you *don't* necessarily focus on the finish line; instead, you focus on where you are at that moment. Checking in with your body, breath, and mind, you pay attention to taking the next step.

There are two key components to marathon success:

Preparation: the proper equipment, nutrition and fuel, water (over time), sleep, hours of practice, etc.

Pacing Yourself: taking things steady. If you push to hit a 4-minute mile with 20 miles remaining, you'll likely putter out before the finish line. You need periodic food and water and a steady pace to finish the race.

Family life goes at a rapid pace. The sheer volume of responsibilities is enormous. Success—and sanity—rely on taking a marathon view. After all, parenting is a marathon, not a sprint. It's a life-long event that requires endurance, attention, commit-

> Don't underestimate the role of endurance in parenting.

ment, and the ongoing awareness that you're in it for the long haul. The sooner you learn to pace yourself, the better for everyone.

Chances are you didn't begin parenting thinking about the importance of a steady pace. Theoretically you knew you were in it for the duration, but before you had kids, you had no idea what that meant! And that was before you discovered your kids had complex needs.

I often say to my clients, "you can do it all, just not at the same time." This awareness—giving yourself permission to focus on incremental change—is positively liberating. Call it what you want—self-care, balance, consciousness, prioritizing—it all comes down to learning to pace yourself.

That means:

- taking the long view;
- accepting that life is a process, not a destination;
- letting go of the need for everything to happen when it "should;"
- allowing kids to develop at their pace, not rushing them to grow up before they're ready;
- accepting that you deserve to take care of yourself too;
- thinking through the next decision, instead of searching for the "right" answer;
- allowing for flexibility, because life changes on a dime;
- letting go of competition and focusing on what's important for your kids; and
- planning for the future while still allowing for change.

Don't underestimate the role of endurance in parenting. The physical challenges—sleeplessness, stress, carrying, and lifting—are enough to keep us fit or age us exponentially. But it's the emotional challenges that keep us up at night. The marathon view can help with this burden, freeing you up from trying to make everything okay forever, and inviting you to focus on next steps for improvement.

Strategy: Take Aim

On a group-coaching call, Janel celebrated that she finally "got" the strategy of Taking Aim. She was working on getting her 7-year-old son to get dressed by himself before school, and she admitted she hadn't believed he could do it independently. Then she repeated, "just one thing," reminding him (and herself) of the goal. Within about a week, he came downstairs dressed and ready for school. She was crying and laughing at the same time.

If you're wondering *how* to take the marathon view without feeling constantly stressed out, start with step 1 of the Impact Model: Take Aim. Instead of trying to do everything, target one challenge at a time, get specific, and get results. You can take aim on either of two levels:

Macro: Look at the big picture and identify a general area that you want to see improved, such as logistics at home at the start of a school year or relationships later in the year.

Micro: Tackle daily concerns, narrowing in on a single focus as specifically as possible. For example, it takes many steps to get from the pillow to the bus stop or carpool. To improve mornings, target the *first* specific behavior you want to see changed, such as waking up, getting out of bed, getting dressed, brushing teeth, or eating breakfast.

If you're thinking "Choose one? But there are so many things I want to take care of!" you're not alone. When there's considerable room for improvement, choosing is difficult. And truly, it almost doesn't matter where you start. Target something you feel will lighten a burden or relieve some pain for you or your child. And yes, it's absolutely acceptable to start by taking aim on something that is making you bug-nuts. Relieving your stress will lighten the load for the whole family.

Ask yourself, "What's the change I want to see?" Depending on your child's progress, focus on that for a day, a week, a month, or longer. In group coaching, we guide parents to Take Aim twice a month. Sometimes they'll choose a new topic for each call; other times, they'll choose the same issue multiple times, taking the time to Rinse and Repeat (Chapter 12) so the change will last.

Cultivating independence happens in baby steps. When we focus on one change at a time, we avoid overwhelm, increase consistency, and get results—for us and our kids. It also allows everyone to experience success, which breeds more success. Taking Aim allows us to help kids increase independence in one area while we scaffold them in others.

For example, if we want kids to get out of bed in the mornings when the alarm goes off, we might continue to provide support the rest of the morning, navigating the hot spots while they focus on getting out of bed independently. Here's the beauty: when one area starts to improve, it cascades into others. Once your child feels successful getting out of bed, they might start brushing their teeth without reminder, as well. You'll see the progress more clearly when you focus on improving one thing at a time.

When a new parent in our private Facebook group asked for advice, a mom from England replied: "Take aim. Just pick one thing at a time to focus on. Otherwise it's so overwhelming. My 10-year-old was diagnosed with combined type ADHD last year. I thought we'd never get out of the dark and challenging place. Almost a year later, it's amazing to see how far we've come."

Say No to Gremlins

As adults, we are alert to cyber-bullying, road rage, and workplace anger management. Bullying starts in childhood and persists throughout our lives. But the worst bullies, by far, are the ones who live inside us. They're the hardest to avoid—and the *only* ones we have the power to change.

We all have an inner voice that's not helpful or supportive. Known in the coaching world as the "inner critic," "saboteur," "gremlin," or "ogre," these internal messengers create mischief in our heads. The gremlin points out everything we're doing wrong and tells us that we can't do anything right. It tries to prevent us from changing anything, in any way—even for the better. Its mission is to maintain the status quo.

> You can change a bully's behavior when that bully is you.

Gremlins can be loud and annoying or softspoken and insidious. Though they sound convincing, they don't speak the truth. They rely on our buy in for their power, but we don't have to give it to them.

My primary gremlin's name is Prudence, and she's a cold, calculating shrew masquerading as a warm, loving, professional Jewish mother. She'd like me to think she's guiding me with the wisdom of Ruth Bader Ginsberg, but I know she's really the voice of Dolores Umbridge. I confess that I used to give Prudence free reign to make me feel terrible about myself. I would never speak to my friends or family the way I let her speak to me.

Do you ever say things to yourself like, "I'm such an idiot," "how could I have been so stupid?," "what was I thinking!?," "I can't do anything right," "there's no way I can do that," or "why would they want me, anyway?"

Those are your gremlins hard at work.

Of course, the bully does not act alone. Like Malfoy has his goons in *Harry Potter*, the internal bully has the world of popular culture—television, movies, magazines, and social media—to protect and energize it. We get messages that we should be thinner, smoother, smarter, and/or sexier. Our gremlins cruelly turn these social images on us. They reinforce all of the world's misleading "shoulds" (see Chapter 1).

I taught my kids to recognize their gremlin voices, and even gave them little gremlin finger-puppets to squeeze in their pockets when they started to feel bad about themselves. I've had adult clients put their gremlin finger-puppets on refrigerator magnets and radio controls in the car. Anything to externalize and expose them for the menaces they can be.

HOW TO TAME THE BULLY WITHIN

Pay attention to the messages you tell yourself. If you hear yourself saying things you'd never say to someone you love, ask yourself, "Is that true?" Don't let your bully get away with speaking lies and pretending they're facts.

Fail forward (see Chapter 8). Cut yourself some slack and learn from your mistakes without making yourself "bad."

Accept life's "whoops" factor. Stop making excuses or blaming others for mistakes; they happen. Owning your mistakes will earn respect from others and help you stand up to your gremlins with confidence.

The challenge with gremlins is that they have the inside scoop. They know how to push our buttons better than anyone, and how to use them at just that weak moment when they'll hit a vulnerable spot. But you can change a bully's behavior when that bully is you. When you do, you'll teach your children to do the same. *That's* the best way to stand up to a bully!

Say Yes to What's Most Important

I was once so worried that my kids wouldn't learn to manage the basics of their lives that I tried to capture everything they needed to do, every day, from Sun-up to Sun-down, in one "simple" reward chart. It was the pinnacle of my trying to do it all. In hindsight, it was an absurd attempt to try to control everything (see Chapter 10).

The chart was ridiculously complicated—they earned two points for this, lost a point for that. It was more than I could keep track of, and a whole lot more than anyone could handle. My need to tackle every problem at once left me, my husband, and my kids feeling overwhelmed and discouraged.

In theory, if I had captured all the things that I thought were important as a quiet guideline for myself to tackle one at a time, it could have been useful. But as a daily task list, it stressed out the whole family. I didn't understand

Everything: Earn & Lose

EARNING POINTS

Task	Points	Mon	Tue	Wed	Thu	Fri	Sat	Sun
Morning Routine								
Out of Bed by 6:45am	2							
Make Bed & Lights Out	2							
Downstairs by 7:05	2							
Take Vitamins @ Bfast	2							
Glass of water @ Bfast	1							
Ready to Walk @ 7:40am	2							
Feed the Dog (Josh)	1							
Nose Wash, Sprays and Steam	5							
After-School Routine								
Unload Backpack/Look at Planner	1							
Lunchbox unpacked (fridge & dishwashe	2							
Get a Snack	1							
Cup of water	1							
Start homework without reminder	1							
Homework put away when done (Josh)	1							
Hang coats on hooks & shoes away	2							
Put backpacks where they belong	1							
Nose Wash, Sprays and Steam	5							
Check Planner for Homework	2							
Mealtime Routine								
Stay at Table (Josh)	1							
Try new food	1							
Excuse self	1							
Clear Plate & to Dishwasher	1							
Take Trash out after meal, as needed	1							
Clearing Parents' Plates	1							
Evening Routine								
Take Vitamins (if forgotten in a.m.)	1							
Bed on time (Josh: 8; syd: 9; Bec: 10)	1							
Read to self for 15/20 min	2							
Lights out (Josh: 8:30; syd: 9:30; B 10)	1							
Ten Minute Clean up (table, HW, room)	3							
Nose Wash, Sprays and Steam	5							
Pack Backpacks/Homework away	1							
Weekly Routines								
Exercise (3-4x) (1 ea; 5 for 4)	1							
Practice Instruments (3-4x) (1 ea; 5 fo	1							
Clean Cubbies/empty Basket (noon Sun	3							
Put Away Laundry (by Fri)	3							
Return bucket to laundry rm by mon a.	1							
Clean Dog's ears	2							
Wash Dog	2							
Recycling/Trash Down the Hill	1							
Recycling/Trash containers up the hill	1							
Fill in Next Week's Planner	2							
Miscellaneous Points--Discretionary								
Wash cars	5							
Vacuum Cars	5							
Mow the Lawn	5							
Blow the Leaves	5							
Do own Laundry	4							
Take Laundry upstairs	1							
Pick up Sticks and rocks (lawn)	2							

LOSING POINTS

Task	Points	Mon	Tue	Wed	Thu	Fri	Sat	Sun
Morning Routine								
Downstairs after 7:15am	-5							
Shoes not on before leaving	-2							
Leave lunch at home	#							
Leave lunch at home & have delivered	#							
Feed self before dog (Josh)	-2							
After-School Routine								
Lunchbox NOT cleared	-3							
Coats not on hooks	-2							
Mealtime Routine								
Leave Table without clearing	-1							
Not Taking Vitamins all day	-2							
No polite bite	-1							
Evening Routine								
More than 15 min late (Josh)	-3							
More than 30 min late (Syd)(Bec)	-3							
Homework not put away/backpack unre	-3							
Weekly Routines								
Walk by laundry at bottom of stairs	-3							
Don't clean cubbies/basket	-5							
Kat's Water Empty (Syd)	-2							
Clothes not away by Sun 5:00	-5							
Laundry basket not down by Mon	-1							
Miscellaneous Points--Discretionary								
"I was just..."	-1							
"I know" without listening	-1							
"wait...wait...wait..."	-1							
Leaving stuff lying around (basket)	-5							
Arguing when asked to do family chore	-5							
Leaving computer light on	-2							
Not logging out of Homework computer	-2							
Not throwing out trash/Cleaning up after	-2							
Screaming at parent/adult (-2 to -5)								
Hitting, kicking, biting (-2 to -5)								
Tantrums/meltdowns (-2 to -5)								

how important it was to simplify what was on my kids' plates, so they could figure out where to focus. Some things needed to wait.

When our kids are babies, we want them to be happy and healthy, which is relatively easy to accomplish. As they grow older, the stakes get higher. Everything from the moment they awaken to the time they go to sleep represents their future. We lose sight of our deep desire for them to be healthy and happy.

It's a tall order to expect all that we want from them at once. We look to outcomes, such as finished homework, good grades, and completed chores. We establish measures of success, such as doing well in school, making and keeping good friends, and being obedient, respectful, and considerate. We want it all—now.

For your child's long-term health and happiness, start small. Focus on the next hurdle instead of the long race. As you embrace the marathon, take aim to quiet the gremlin voices and focus on what's absolutely most important for your child's growth and development. That means deciding for yourself (and your child) what's most important—next.

Write yourself a simple question on a sticky note to help you clarify your priorities; for example, "What's most important here?" or "What's my priority in this moment?" Keep it where you can see it—on the refrigerator, over the kitchen desk, or in your underwear drawer. When you find yourself getting aggravated at one more incomplete task, take a breath and ask yourself the question.

Is your priority to get kids through high school to college? Is it to prepare them for whatever direction their life takes? Is it about individual achievements or relationships? Sometimes you may discover that it's important that the trash goes out immediately—and there's your answer. Or you may discover that, after a rough day, your child is finally getting something done on their homework and you don't want to interrupt.

> For your child's long-term health and happiness, start small. Focus on the next hurdle instead of the long race.

In any given moment, there are dozens of expectations that you have for your child, all important in the long run. But in the short term, it helps immensely to prioritize, weaving a fabric of successes over the long term. Remember that all things can be accomplished over time. Prioritizing, based on what's most important to you, prevents the "stuff" of life from becoming a higher priority than the people in it.

Self-Talk: Really, Put on Your Oxygen Mask First

Years ago, child and family therapist David Alexander brought a large, broken rubber band to a presentation for parents. It had been circling large files in an attic somewhere, dry and brittle after being stretched out for too long. Eventually even the most pliable rubber band will lose its elasticity if it's kept stretched thin. He explained the metaphor: Parents need to release the tension once in a while so that we don't snap.

In theory, you know you have to take care of yourself to meet the needs of your children. But believing that is difficult for many of us. However, self-care is not just some luxury afforded other parents. Success starts with how you talk to yourself and think about it.

This is going to sound impossible to some of you. To be completely honest, I still struggle with this every day. I'm much more focused on the needs of my family or my work than my own needs. But when I allow myself to get burnt out, everyone suffers.

The Impact Model is circled in self-care because it's essential to everything in this book. Like putting on your oxygen mask first on an airplane, so that you can assist others in need, you must put yourself on your priority list, not just in theory but in practice. This approach works better when you're a healthy part of the equation. Pacing yourself for the long haul is hard to do if you're passed out on the floor from lack of oxygen.

> Kids with chronic issues need to learn to consciously take care of themselves, and your self-care models positive self-management.

Not convinced? Imagine if it was important to get (at least some of) your needs met. Getting enough sleep (no, I'm not joking), learning to set limits for yourself, or date nights with partners or friends.

If you actually turn some attention to keeping yourself nourished, how will that impact your family? Could you be replenished enough to handle the meltdown when your child is worried that they can't do a math assignment? Could you be calm enough to not take the bait when your teen starts pushing your buttons?

And what about the indirect impact on them? Kids with chronic issues need to learn to consciously take care of themselves, and your self-care models positive self-management. As experiential learners, when they see you take care of yourself, they're more likely to follow suit eventually. "Do as I say, not as I do" doesn't work with these kids. They'll learn by seeing it in action.

One mom in our community stopped exercising when she took a full-time job because she felt guilty for spending less time at home. As her irritability grew, she thought the job was the problem. Then her kids asked her to start working out again, nearly begging her to return to her self-care routine.

Similarly, when my husband started to exercise more regularly, the kids saw him enjoy it and challenge himself—and they got the message. They started to do the same on their own, and at least two of them became engaged athletes. They may wax and wane in how they exercise in their lives, but its importance to them is clear. I think it's directly related to my husband's modeling something he was doing for himself.

Taking better care of yourself will help you better focus on the needs of your family. If you want to be able to assist others in need, you have to keep yourself fueled.

Questions for Self-Discovery

- Grab your journal or notebook and list everything that's adding to your load. Keep going. Get it out!
- How can a Marathon View help you?
- What's one macro area, and three micro areas inside it, where you might want to Take Aim? Choose one to start.
- What do your gremlin voices say to you?
- What's most important to you as a parent?
- List the ways you tell yourself that self-care is not important. (Go back to your journal or notebook if you need to.) Now, next to each of them, reframe those messages in a way that's more helpful.

LINDA'S STORY

The first time I spoke with Linda, she called from her closet. Because she was constantly in a state of fight or flight, she stayed late at the office most days, and then she retreated to her closet when she got home, figuring it was better than buying a one-way ticket out of town (which she secretly wanted). She told me about a huge blow-up from a few nights before, an event that finally led her to schedule a Sanity Session. The sheetrock could be repaired, she said, but the damage from the things she'd said—words she could never take back—would last forever. She was clear, maybe for the first time, that although her son was not blameless, her inability to control herself was exacerbating things. She wanted to stop the chaos that was swirling around her constantly and learn to manage things better. I assured her that although we can't always control what happens, I could help her learn to respond to what happens with more grace and respect.

Bottom Line: Linda was seriously concerned about the damage caused by words she could never take back. Her inability to control herself wasn't helping. In fact, it was making things worse.

CHAPTER 6

"Why Can't They Just . . . ?"

No One Knows Your Child Better Than You Do

"Understanding the nature of the situation makes it much easier to transform it." —THICH NHAT HANH

"Why Can't They Just . . . "

No matter how well-meaning they are, many loved ones and caring friends will never fully grasp the reality of your life. It's so much more complicated than it appears on the surface!

Complex issues, such as ADHD, anxiety, autism, LD, and related challenges, look different for every person facing them. They're not tangible (like blood sugar numbers) or visible (like broken bones). They creep into every crack and crevice of daily life.

Parents spend years trying to get a basic understanding so we can guide our kids through the labyrinth of their complex brains. But we secretly battle an internal conflict: Sometimes we ourselves struggle to accept that our kids' issues are real.

- It's scary that our kids are not on par, developmentally, with their peers.
- It's infuriating that we feel like broken records, constantly directing and redirecting.
- It's maddening that our otherwise sweet kid speaks to their siblings, or to us, in ways that would make a sailor blush.

When we get frustrated or annoyed, exhausted or overwhelmed, we don't consider that there's a legitimate reason why our kids aren't doing what's expected of them. We just want them to be "typical" for long enough to give us a break.

> We just want them to be "typical" for long enough to give us a break.

So, when well-meaning people say "If you would just . . . " and suggest using discipline, holding them accountable, setting a clear limit, or "not letting them talk to you like that," we internalize these comments and feel ineffective.

And we unwittingly do the same to our kids. As a client of mine writes, "what I really wanted was for [my son] to 'just' hand in his homework, 'just' not get so emotional, 'just' follow simple directions, 'just,' well, you can fill in the blanks."

How often do you wonder how on Earth something happened, only to have a glimmer of recognition? "Oh yeah, that was impulsive!" or "Yup, that kid got distracted!" or "Wow, she doesn't even remember that conversation."

On one level, you know why your kid can't just remember to put clothes in the laundry or stop overreacting or picking fights with a teasing sibling. Various aspects of executive function are lagging behind, and they aren't performing appropriately for their chronological age (see Chapter 7).

And yet, sometimes it takes a while to grasp the depth of it. Even when they know their kids are developmentally delayed in theory, parents often say things such as:

- "I know he has anxiety, but it's unacceptable that he doesn't do what I ask when I give him a direction."
- "Why do they jump on the couch right after I tell them not to?"
- "Why is he so sensitive?"
- "Why doesn't she tell me what's going on?"
- "I just realized that his ADHD is really at the cause of all of this. You've been telling me for two years, but I think it's just sinking in."
- "Why do I have to repeat myself?"
- "Why doesn't he turn in his homework if he's actually done it?"

"Why," we ask. "Why didn't you . . . ?" "Why don't you . . . ?" "Why can't they just . . . ?" These questions express powerlessness, wreaking havoc for us and for them. We believe they'll guide us to answers. Instead, the word *why* is a trigger that fuels our frustration, escalates a situation, and puts others on the defensive. "Why can't you just . . ." locks our kids into a perpetual cycle of failure, and it locks us into a victim state where things are being done to us.

Adults who also have complex brains struggle with this too. We know we forget things or struggle with time management. But we don't want our kids to suffer the way we have, so sometimes we're even harder on them, holding them to impossible standards. Instead of saying, "Why can't they just," we shift to "If they would just." The result is the same.

Coach's Reframe: Is It Naughty or Neurological?

You walk in at 5:30 pm after a long day at work and 30 minutes of unexpected traffic. Now you have to get dinner going and homework done. Your youngest needs a bath before dinner, or you'll never get everyone ready for bedtime. You ask your 14-year-old (who has ADHD and anxiety) to boil a pot of water while you get your 6-year-old into a bath. More than anything, you want your child to say, "Sure, Mom. Anything else I can do?" Instead, your son screams, "I can't do that! I've got so much homework it's not even funny. You have no idea how much math I've got—our teacher hates us! And my Lit paper turns out to be due tomorrow. They never told us! There's no way!"

You're closer to boiling than that pot of water. You want to scream: "You rotten kid, do you know what kind of day I've had? I'm not asking you to make dinner, which you should be able to do by your age, anyway. It's just a pot of water!"

Instead of blowing your fuse, you take a deep breath, let it out, and ask yourself: "Is It Naughty or Neurological?" What's really going on? Your son struggles with intense emotions, which escalated when he realized he didn't plan ahead, and writing is so difficult for him. He's stuck in overwhelm, impulsively lashing out because he's been holding it in all day. Your child is struggling, and you're a safe place for him to let it out.

I learned to ask this question from Dr. Kathleen Platzman circa 2002, and I've been using it ever since. Any time you're tempted to ask yourself "why can't they just . . . ?", replace it with "Is it naughty or neurological?"

A simple request to boil a pot of water involves a whole host of executive functions. If you understand the neurological connection, you may still get frustrated, but you'll be more supportive than if you think they're being rude. For example, you might:

Acknowledge what's going on so your child can recognize it. ("Wow, you sound really upset. I guess you're feeling stressed by all that work.")

Show compassion. ("I hate it when I'm feeling like there's not enough time. I'm feeling like that, too, so I can relate.")

Modify or negotiate, giving your child some control. ("I didn't realize you have so much on your plate too—if you get the water started, I'll have more time to help with your paper tonight. Will that work? We'll get through it together!")

The brain is ultimately responsible for all behaviors, and executive function governs every aspect of life—thoughts, feelings, and actions. Understanding the simple fact that there's often a neurological explanation for any behavior can be liberating. It releases you from a tendency to blame and judge and connects you to compassion and understanding.

Sure, sometimes kids are mischievous or naughty. If it's naughty and you put systems in place to correct the behavior, it's likely to shift. But if it's neurological, chances are that all the deterrents in the world will not change the behavior.

> If it's neurological, chances are that all the deterrents in the world will not change the behavior.

In the next few chapters, I'll introduce strategies and tactics to help you respond effectively as you identify underlying neurological causes of difficult behaviors. Once you acknowledge that your child is struggling with something, the next step is to take what a client of mine calls "the curiosity approach."

Strategy: Don't Get Furious, Get Curious (Before You Plan)

I know they say that curiosity kills the cat, but what if a parent's *lack of curiosity* actually creates a danger zone for kids?

Even with reasonable explanations, our kids' behaviors can make it unbelievably hard to cope. We get frustrated, scared, angry, overwhelmed, and hopeless. Parents with robust executive function skills want nothing more than a good plan, while those of us with our own executive function challenges may see *plan* as a four-letter-word. Either way, we all want a clear path forward, and curiosity is your path—it paves the way to more effective planning and problem solving.

Whenever you start to judge anyone's behavior (not just your kids), just notice that. Take a breath and remind yourself to get curious. Ask yourself questions such as "what's going on here?" or "what's motivating them?" or "what might be happening to lead to that behavior?" Curiosity can shift your focus from "why are they doing that?" to "I wonder what they're going through." It shifts your mindset from "why can't they just . . . " to "is it naughty or neurological?"

Curiosity is the chief tool to use in step 2 of the Impact Model. After taking aim on a change you want to see (see Chapter 5), use curiosity to start collecting information or getting educated about what's going on. A little detective work can help you look at things from a range of perspectives and uncover underlying motivations and obstacles. What's your perspective? How is your child experiencing it? What about the school or other members of the family? Use the acronym WIGO to ask yourself What Is Going On?

In each of the next four chapters, I'll introduce four contexts to consider when putting together a plan to tackle any dilemma. Whenever you get confused, don't know what to say, or cannot believe how someone is acting, get curious using these lenses and see what becomes possible:

Activating the Brain: Most behaviors are influenced by what's happening in the body and the brain, chemically, and this is true for both complex kids and overwhelmed, stressed parents. Whether you activate the brain through exercise, nutrition, sleep, medication, meditation, coaching, or something else, enhancing its ability to work as effectively as possible is essential to any plan.

Positivity: Complex kids are consistently dropping, losing, breaking or forgetting things, and getting corrected from morning to night—which parents often do without even realizing it. Maintaining your relationship and their self-esteem, despite frequent mistakes and redirections, is key. Look for your kids' potential and empower them to buy into their own success by focusing on what's possible.

Shifting Expectations: You have every reason to set high expectations for your kids. The trick is to do it in a developmentally appropriate way. Because complex kids are about 3 to 5 years (roughly 30%) behind their same-age peers in some aspects of their development, setting expectations realistically allows them to feel successful regardless of their age. Shifting expectations is *not* settling for "less" or "lowering" expectations.

Creating Systems and Structures Effectively: The routines and processes we use to make improvements and manage our lives are most effective when developed in the context of Activating the Brain, Positivity, and Shifted Expectations. Systems and structures are not an end goal—they are a means to help us with self-management, self-regulation, and achieving personal success.

Curiosity offers an opportunity to support your kids, ultimately increasing their success and responsibility by creating plans that work in real life.

Say No to the Shame and Blame Game

We don't want our kids to feel bad about themselves, but we're desperate for them to take responsibility for their actions, or to feel grateful for all that we're doing for them. So, we begin to point fingers, even though we don't mean to shame or blame them.

> We want to help our kids see that they're not bad, they're struggling—and we can help them with that.

Meanwhile, our kids don't want to lie or disappoint us, but as they begin to feel "naughty" for behaviors that are actually neurological, they develop feelings of shame and embarrassment. It's a vicious cycle.

Defensiveness and offensiveness abound in equal measure in the homes of complex kids. Kids of all ages want to be seen as "good," but when they struggle with that, they often end up seeing themselves as "bad." So, either they get aggressive (sometimes even abusive), or they become defensive and avoid taking responsibility. Then their reactions reinforce your deepest concerns, and you're caught in an endless loop of the Shame and Blame Game.

This is one of the most common scenarios I encounter in my practice (regardless of a kids' age or diagnoses). For example it can be hard to accept that kids don't avoid work just to be rude, difficult, or disrespectful. In fact these behaviors have nothing to do with whether they respect or appreciate us. If they don't have a mechanism to get themselves activated, that can be embarrassing for them. They certainly don't need us reminding them, much less making them feel bad about it.

Even the best parents have some unhealthy patterns that could be improved and ways of communicating that could be more supportive. To change oppositional communication patterns, even with older kids:

PART TWO

1. Notice when shame and blame crop up in your words, tone of voice, or assumptions, and try to stop them in their tracks. More than likely, they're interfering with your ability to build and maintain a trusting relationship and with your child's ability to take responsibility.

2. If you find yourself feeling embarrassed or worried about what others might think about you or your child, those are feelings of shame, too. Get some support (from a coach, a therapist, or a friend) to set appropriate expectations based on what your child needs, not what others think, so you can empower your kid to reach their full potential.

3. If reading this is triggering guilt or shame for you, please reread Chapter 2, especially "Up Until Now" and "Put the Stick Down." Seek support and put effort into managing your own triggers so you can be fully present for your kids.

4. If you have a child who tends to be extremely defensive or lies a lot (a kind of defensive dishonesty), chances are they have a lot of feelings of shame that they are not yet navigating well; or they're feeling blamed, even if you aren't communicating that consciously. Use nonjudgmental, matter-of-fact language to remove the unintentional shame they're absorbing.

Bottom line: We want to hold our kids accountable for their behaviors, without feeling that they're somehow morally bankrupt. We want to distinguish between a bad behavior and a bad kid. And we want to help our kids see that they're not bad, they're struggling—and we can help them with that.

Say Yes to a Disability Perspective

"The important thing is to see and encourage potential." —The Upside

If your child were in a wheelchair, you wouldn't put them at the bottom of a flight of stairs and tell them to run up to the top. To reach the top, you'd expect it to take time and effort—perhaps using their arms or maybe setting up a pulley system. Their achievement in reaching the top would be sweet for their struggle, and you'd likely celebrate heartily. Similarly when a child has anxiety, speaking to a teacher or spending the night at a friend's might be an enormous step for them. Instead of telling them that they have nothing to worry about, you might acknowledge their concerns and help them devise a plan to achieve their goal with your support.

Some kids have medical reasons that impair them from using parts of their bodies. Our kids have medical reasons that delay the development of essential executive function skills in their brains. I want to encourage you to apply a disability perspective to your child's emotional, social, and organizational development.

Many parents resist the idea that their kids have a disability, as I did for many years. I didn't want it to be true. I wanted them to be "normal" or "typical." I wanted them to fit in. I wanted things to be easy for them—and for me.

Parents tell me that they don't want to "label" their child's challenges because they don't want the label itself to become a crutch. They want their child to learn to navigate life, so they don't want to give them excuses. But when a kid needs crutches, they need crutches. We expect something different from them in specific ways for a time, and we support them in ways that they need—usually not for long. But if they don't take the weight off of that broken leg, it might not heal well, and then they *might* need the crutches forever.

A disability perspective acknowledges that there's a reason our kids can't do what's asked of them—yet. If we don't lighten the load while our kids' brains are catching up, they may never acquire the skills they need to learn.

Kids' challenges show up in all aspects of life and learning: managing emotions, organization, procrastination, following instructions, going to a restaurant, and the like. They may need reminders to get started on their homework, or help organizing their backpack. Rather than asking them to clean their room, you might start by focusing on one shelf or drawer. With support, they'll get there over time. But when kids are less mature than their same-aged peers, or not as skilled at self-management, we must make sure we're not telling them to hop out of the wheelchair and run up the stairs.

As a parent, this perspective allows you to advocate and educate your child based on your child's current capacity.

It helps to:

- Let go of how others see you as a parent and focus on your child.
- Stop constantly comparing kids to their same-aged peers and set realistic expectations based on their developmental age.
- Take aim consciously, deliberately deciding what's appropriate to let go (for now).
- Advocate in school for reasonable, developmentally appropriate accommodations and modifications.
- Improve communication by clarifying what's expected of kids so they can respond successfully.

We help complex kids most when we recognize, embrace, and accept them for who they are—for their very humanness—and teach them to do the same. They are children, teens, and young adults, struggling to fulfill the world's expectations in life and learning. When we shed outdated notions of perfectionism that unwittingly leave kids feeling broken and worthless, we empower them to embrace and understand themselves.

Whatever the challenge, a disability perspective offers an opportunity to shift our expectations with an emphasis on what kids *can* do, so we can help children learn to be successful based on where they are developmentally, one skill at a time.

Self-Talk: Responding Instead of Reacting

Remember the family dinner scene in the 2015 movie *Inside Out*? As the conversation gets more uncomfortable and emotions get stirred up, the daughter, who is trying to hold it together, finally slams her hands on the table in frustration, yelling "Just shut up!" Though she's not asking calmly, she is trying to get a break to reclaim her brain. Instead of giving her space and slowing things down, the dad yells, "That's it, go to your room!"

It's considered one of the best scenes from that inspiring movie, probably because it captures a family dynamic that most of us recognize. We all—parents and kids—have reacted when triggered, escalating the situation (with tears, fuming, empty threats, harsh punishments, or even holes in walls). But helping kids manage their reactivity starts with learning to manage our own.

> You can't control what happens; you can only control how you *respond* to what happens.

When people recognize the need to calm themselves down, that's a healthy response, whatever their age. The dad in *Inside Out* failed to recognize that his daughter was trying to get a handle on her difficult emotions. As a result, his reactivity prevented anyone from calming things down so they could respond differently.

You can't control what happens; you can only control how you *respond* to what happens. When you enter into conversation with yourself, you can start to get a handle on your own reactivity.

COACH YOURSELF TO RESPOND WITHOUT REACTING

What are your key triggers? Identify what pushes your buttons despite your best intentions. What's really causing your aggravation? Are you triggered by rushing, being late, kids talking back or speaking crudely, disrespect, or looking at grades online?

What are the thoughts/feelings behind the triggers? A parent might feel guilt, frustration, and overwhelm before opening the online grading portal, thinking, "He's probably missing 17 assignments, it'll be terrible, and I'll have screwed up because I'm not more on top of it." A parent who hates to be late might think, "The teacher is going to think I don't care and she's not going to want to help." Or a parent who wants their child to learn from them might think, "My son has absolutely no respect for me and doesn't care what I think."

What is a more supportive thought? These stories we tell ourselves may have a shred of truth—maybe you screwed up, or the teacher will judge you, or your child doesn't respect you. But they're taken out of proportion and distorted by our gremlins (see Chapter 5). So, choose a helpful and supportive message that you can believe that helps you calm down. It could be true that you're doing the best you can, that the teacher will understand you're trying, or that your child has immense respect for you but can't show it when he's upset.

Once you start to manage your reactivity, you'll help your kids do the same. Although it's not realistic to stop them from ever getting triggered, reducing the intensity and frequency *is* possible. When you hear a teenager scream something like, "I'm sorry I'm yelling right now, I'm just really frustrated and I don't know why," you have done your job well.

Working on triggers together as a family is actually quite powerful too. If it's expected that everyone could lose it occasionally, and you support each other to get a handle on things when that happens, it becomes a partnership. Imagine your kid saying, "I'm triggered, give me 5 minutes and I'll come back."

Understanding triggers helps people know when they need a break and how to respond without so much reactivity. According to Dr. Russell Barkley, adults with ADHD are more likely to lose jobs for losing their temper than not turning in a project. So, responding instead of reacting is an essential life skill—one of the greatest gifts you can give yourself, your kids, and your precious relationships.

Questions for Self-Discovery

- When do you fall into the "why can't they just . . . " trap?
- What's different when you ask, "is it naughty or neurological?"
- What makes you curious?
- What blame or shame are you ready to let go?
- What behavior(s) could benefit from a disability perspective?
- Which reaction can you shift to become more responsive?

HENRY'S STORY

"I know my son doesn't have one of those buttons you talk about, but I just don't know what else to do," Henry wrote. "I tell him to do something, he says he's going to do it, and then he doesn't. And I just don't know how to get him to do it. I don't want to spend the rest of my life taking care of him. I was planning to retire, but now it looks like I never will." Henry had started Sanity School®, so he understood that his son Jackson had executive function challenges and was not purposefully messing up; but he feared Jackson would never become independent because he didn't follow directions. As Henry talked with Jackson about what was important to him, and helped Jackson understand his motivators, Henry shifted his approach. He stopped barking orders and began to encourage Jackson to gradually take ownership of his actions.

Bottom Line: "I know my son doesn't have one of those buttons you talk about, but I just don't know what else to do. I tell him to do something, he says he's going to do it, and then he doesn't."

CHAPTER 7

"My Kid's Just Not Motivated"

How to Get Your Kids to . . . [Fill in the Blank]

> "The most effective way to show compassion to another is to listen, rather than talk." —THICH NHAT HANH

Kids Don't Have a "Just Get It Done" Button

Some people are motivated by a list of what needs to be done. Sometimes they'll even write something they've done just so they can check it off. They thrive on a feeling of accomplishment and completion and are eager to do what's expected of them, either because someone else expects it or because they want to do it for themselves. A sense of obligation, or expectation, is enough to get them moving—and stuff gets done.

Chances are, that doesn't describe your child (and possibly not you).

Our kids are typically not motivated by crossing things off a list, doing what's expected of them, or doing what's good for them. By puberty, they're generally no longer sufficiently motivated by making us happy either. Even when they agree to do something we want, that may not be enough stimulation for them to get it done. They need another way to get their brains activated.

In other words, people who struggle with executive function typically don't have a "just get it done" button.

Some people can just buckle down and get something done because their brains are wired to make that happen. The chemicals in their brain will fire and receive information appropriately on command. If you're one of those

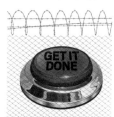

BRAIN SCIENCE SIMPLIFIED

The brain sends messages through chemical reactions that help us think, feel, or act. Neurotransmitters, chemicals that transmit signals through neurons, are released and let parts of the brain communicate with each other. Due to reduced levels of transmitters, such as dopamine, serotonin, or norepinephrine, kids with anxiety, depression, ADHD, or executive function challenges don't always have the brain chemistry necessary to make something happen without external forces stepping in to help.

people, it may be hard to understand that it's not that simple for everyone. When you're faced with something you don't want to do, you simply press an imaginary "just get it done" button, and *voila*, you can make it happen.

But with complex brains that are differently wired, a delayed or compromised executive function system makes it feel like there's barbed wire in front of your personal "get it done" button. You don't have the internal controls needed to remember what you want or don't want to do, and when; your ability to self-regulate is compromised.

If you're not genuinely interested or engaged (and sometimes, even when you are), it's extremely difficult to initiate, sustain, or complete any given action. It's like walking through the poppy fields in the *Wizard of Oz*. At first it's exciting and looks easy enough, and you set out to cross the field with the best of intentions. But pretty soon you're succumbing to the soporific effects of the poppies; and before you know it, you've lost sight of the task and are taken over by a nap attack.

It's not that you're lazy or irresponsible. It's that your brain can only fight those poppies for so long without external supports stepping in. To stay the course, you'll need an understanding of what's happening in the brain, clear intention, and some structures in place to help make things happen. As you learn to harness the power of your brain to get it activated, you'll begin to be able to get things done.

Coach's Reframe: Explore Executive Function (Activating the Brain)

Executive function (EF) is a term that parents hear a lot and feel like we're supposed to understand. But to be honest, most of us don't have a clue. I know I didn't for years! That is why the first eBook Diane and I wrote in 2012 was *What the Heck Is Executive Function and Why Should You Care?*

So, let me make it super simple. There are basically two primary parts of the brain involved with getting anything done: the primitive brain (hindbrain) and the frontal lobe (prefrontal cortex).

The primitive brain keeps us alive, releasing adrenaline ("stress" hormone) and telling us to freeze, fight, or flee when in danger. People with a sluggish frontal lobe may overrely on the primitive brain to get things done—such as waiting until the last minute so that the sense of urgency forces the primitive brain into action.

The frontal lobe is where the executive functions reside. It organizes, manages time, and tells us what to think, feel, and do (or not do), enabling a person to decide to do something and follow through to completion. Many complex kids are developmentally delayed in this part of the brain.

EF is an umbrella term for the skills involved with organization and self-management, directing nearly every thought, feeling, or action. If you think of the brain's frontal lobe as the orchestra conductor of the brain, then the players in the orchestra are the different executive functions. If just one player is out of tune, the brain's function will be discordant.

Dr. Thomas Brown, author of *Attention Deficit Disorder* and *Smart but Stuck*, identified six aspects of behavior that people challenged with EF could have difficulty managing. Your kids may be challenged in one area, or in all six. Because getting anything done relies on activating the brain, understanding the six aspects of EF is essential to proactive planning. As you get clear on how different challenges manifest, you can develop strategies to improve your kids' self-regulation.

According to Sheryl Pruitt, author of *Taming the Tiger*, EF challenges manifest in more than 100 childhood conditions, including

- neurological disorders, such as ADHD, anxiety, autism, Tourette syndrome, and depression;
- metabolic diseases, such as phenylketonuria (PKU), celiac disease, Addison's disease, and allergies;
- learning disabilities and other challenges of twice exceptional (2E) kids; and
- stress-related conditions, such as attachment disorder, trauma, and PTSD.

For complex kids, it's not whether you need to activate the brain, it's how. Using any combination of exercise, nutrition, sleep, medication, meditation, coaching, or motivation, understanding EF and consciously engaging the frontal lobe will improve a child's ability to self-regulate.

SIX AREAS OF EXECUTIVE FUNCTION

Task Management (Activation): Organizing, Prioritizing, and Initiating Activity Looks like: has difficulty getting started; procrastinates; knows what needs to be done but is unable to get it done; has difficulty prioritizing and sequencing; fails in time management; does things last minute. Appears to the untrained eye as "lazy."

Attention Management (Focus): Focusing, Sustaining, and Shifting Attention to Tasks Looks like: gets "bored" easily; requires "genuine interest" to sustain focus; distractible; has difficulty discerning what's important to focus on; hyperfocused; gets stuck on something (common with video games); is unable to move off a task.

Energy/Effort Management (Effort): Alertness, Sustaining Effort, Processing Speed Looks like: tires quickly when required to sit quietly; has trouble maintaining alertness; needs steady stimulation or feedback (physical or mental) to stay alert; processes slowly; takes a long time to read and/or write. With hyperactivity: has difficulty slowing down to assure quality work; has trouble regulating body's engine.

Emotion Management: Managing Frustration and Modulating Emotions Looks like: low frustration threshold (short fuse); impatient; has difficulty regulating emotions; oversensitive; responds "inappropriately"; takes things personally; easily "taken over" by emotions.

Information Management (Memory): Using Working Memory and Accessing Recall Looks like: has trouble "holding" some information while working on other information; has trouble with complex math problems and/ or writing; forgets feelings of love and connection when upset; is forgetful.

Action Management: Monitoring and Self-Regulating Action Looks like: hyperactive; impulsive; difficulty deciding when to act or not act; makes inappropriate comments or jokes; confronts friends or family at the wrong time; interrupts or calls out in class; has trouble keeping up with conversation; exhibits "randomness."

PART TWO

Strategy: Understand and Use Motivation

It seems like: "This kid isn't motivated by anything. They only do what they want to do." When you ask what motivates them, you get responses like, "I don't know" or "whatever." It's maddening.

What's really happening: Your kid's brain is seeking stimulation to get going, and it's only "naturally" activated by things they find engaging. Activating the brain can be done with medicine, exercise, and a number of other external structures, but it must be consciously applied.

There are five potential motivators that are like a hidden charm to get activated. Teach kids to identify *which* of these works best for them, because most people aren't easily motivated by all five.

MOTIVATION = P.I.N.C.H.
Play. Humans are inherently motivated by things that are fun, pleasurable, or enjoyable. So, play, creativity, and humor are effective instigators for action. To help a kid get something done, turn it into a game, make a joke, or let them get creative. When possible, tie into other motivators, such as interest, novelty, and competition.

Interest. Because complex brains seek stimulation, "boring" is like kryptonite, while "interesting" ignites a power chamber. Find something compelling to get anything done. Students who do well with engaging teachers or in subjects they find interesting tend to be motivated by interest.

Novelty. Complex brains like change and innovation. Routines work temporarily, but when the novelty wears off, they become boring. Novelty is a likely motivator for students who start a school year strong (new teachers, classmates, schedules), but engagement wanes over time. Because new is interesting, be willing to change systems as needed.

Competition. Building on several other motivators, competition can provide interest, urgency, novelty, and play. Competition usually offers the possibility of a reward and often plays to someone's strengths. It doesn't work for everyone, though. Those who struggle with anxiety can be stressed rather than motivated by competition with themselves of others.

Hurry-Up (Urgency). People who wait until the last minute to get anything done—whether it's starting homework or getting ready to leave the house— use urgency as a motivator. Because the frontal lobe isn't properly stimulated, last minute uses a different part of the brain—the primitive brain—providing the chemical incentive to take action. When not overused, deadlines can be extremely helpful to activate the brain.

To guide kids to understand and use motivation effectively, ask what they like about their favorite activities.

- One kid loved Minecraft because it is a creative (play), non-competitive game he could play with a friend.
- One kid loves games (competition) and is fascinated by strategy (interest).
- One student with dyslexia, anxiety, and ADHD loved math, so her teacher put sudokus in the classroom (play) as a reward for finishing writing.
- One student was motivated by celebration and acknowledgment (play) and new activities (novelty). His teacher acknowledged what he'd already completed before pointing out what was left to be done.

- A student motivated by laughter (play), arousal energy (urgency), and connection with his dad (interest) started waking up happily when his father tickled him awake or invited the dog to jump on the bed.

Accept it: Your kids need motivation to take action. Learn spelling words or math facts while bouncing a basketball, or let students write spelling words with multicolored pens. Make games out of ... *anything*! Sometimes, you might even let them do something fun *before* they get started, such as reading a page of comics before they take out the trash. If it helps them get started, you'll find it might even motivate you!

Say No to Catastrophizing

Do questions like these compete loudly for airtime in your head?

"What if she doesn't do well in school?"
"What if he never makes friends?"
"What if they can't handle a relationship?"
"What if she's still living in my basement when she's 35?"
"What if he ends up addicted or in jail?"
"What if they live a lonely existence?"
"What if they can't hold down a job?"

If so, it's no wonder you feel overwhelmed. "What if . . . " questions can dominate our daytime to-do lists and wake us up in the middle of the night. When we can't clearly see the path ahead for our kids, we catastrophize. We fear for the worst, allowing ourselves to live in a futuristic dystopia.

But when we panic at the thought that our 12-year-old child will live in squalor at 24 because they don't clean up potato chips after watching a movie, it can be paralyzing. It robs us of the joy of parenting, prevents us from steadily guiding our kids, and interferes with our relationships.

> Accept it: Your kids need motivation to take action.

I'm not saying that you have nothing to "worry" about; parenting any child is nerveracking. But, seriously, keep things in perspective and avoid the temptation to jump to conclusions. Just because they didn't get it done today, doesn't mean they'll never learn. When we panic at each missed step, or only fear for the worst, we rob ourselves—and more importantly, our kids—of the opportunity to learn, improve, and ultimately, experience a sense of accomplishment and success.

Instead of fearing forward twenty years, look back three years. Notice improvements in managing frustration, remembering homework, or controlling impulsivity. Take a moment to appreciate all the successes they've enjoyed and the positive memories you've created. They don't have to be monumental achievements to be worthy of recognition; small victories are worth celebrating.

Now, look forward three years, then another three. Where are they likely to be at 27? Will they maintain their current trajectory, and speed it up, because they have you? Look at the small steps you can take this week and this year. Focus on little outcomes. That's how you'll see progress, and that's how you'll be able to start living more in the moment with your kids.

Catastrophic thoughts and fears will derail you from what really needs your attention. In Chapter 9, we'll talk more about developmental delays and setting realistic expectations. For now, look for opportunities to be present, to move forward slowly and steadily from today to tomorrow. Stay focused on understanding their brain and getting clear on how it's best motivated. Take the time to understand what you need to feel calm and well cared for. It's time to manage your own fears, because they're not serving you, and they're not serving your kids.

> It's time to manage your own fears, because they're not serving you and they're not serving your kids.

Say Yes to Ownership as the Best Reward

Have you ever tried to get fit without rewarding your efforts along the way? It doesn't work, does it? You don't wait until you can run a marathon to reward yourself. Instead you reward yourself for going to the gym every day for a week, or for jogging a mile without stopping, or for saying "no" to a yummy dessert.

There's solid research linking reward systems (such as token economies or star charts) to improving outcomes for complex kids. In fact, rewards are probably the most common behavior-management techniques suggested by psychologists, physicians, and other providers. When used well, rewards are an effective tool for motivating *anyone* to do something they want to do. But as Ross Greene says, "Stickers won't help anyone solve any problems or improve their skills." Ownership and investment are fundamental to success.

Rewards focus on positivity; they're a way of catching kids being "good" instead of focusing on "bad" behaviors. They support good behavior in everyone:

- Complex kids tend to respond more favorably to the carrot than to the stick. This may be because they are redirected more frequently and have more opportunity to be wrong, so rewarding them for behaving well is all the more impactful.
- Parents and teachers respond positively to rewards because it's a whole lot more fun than yelling or punishing. This can make a powerful difference for the self-esteem of a child.

But as effective as rewards can be, they don't always work in reality the way they do in theory. Quite often, after putting a reward system in place, parents or teachers of complex kids find themselves disappointed because it's not the magic bullet they expected. They complain that their child may have achieved a goal but didn't create a habit; once the goal is achieved, the old behavior comes back. That's because rewards don't work well in a vacuum. They have to make as much sense to our kids as they do to us!

Rewards don't work when . . .

Kids are scared. Afraid of failure or afraid of success (yes, fear of success is real: "If I do that well, then my parents will expect more from me!"), anxiety can overpower a gold star.

It's not important enough to them. Due to a lack of ownership and buy-in (see Chapter 10), kids don't care enough about a reward because they haven't bought into the desired goals or process.

Rewards do work when . . .

Someone wants something and is willing to work to achieve it. You can offer a kid ten stars for tying his shoes, but if he's not ready to learn to tie his shoes, he'll never reach for them.

Someone wants to achieve lasting change. A teenager who's interested in driving a car might put more effort into getting a driver's license than a teen who is afraid to drive or uninterested in going out with friends.

Motivators are connected to positive rewards. It can improve someone's willingness to work toward a goal.

Rewards don't have to be big, and they don't have to cost money. When Diane's daughter was 9, for example, she was genuinely motivated by being able to choose the radio station on the way to school. But it *is* essential to include a child in the conversation and decision to put a reward system in place. Not only do you want them to buy in to the goal you've set, ideally you want them to be part of identifying what reward they want to earn.

You can empower your child to make great changes, one step at a time, with an effective reward system that they're invested in using. And you'll go from feeling like the bad guy to feeling like the superstar parent you are.

Self-Talk: Know What Feeds You

As a brand new mom, I went out to a baby shower, leaving my baby at home with David. I called after the party, only to find that there was no need to rush home. "Go have a good time," my husband told me. "Take a break."

I didn't know what to do with myself, so I ended up walking around the top floor of a mall crying. I wasn't exactly sad; I was lost. I didn't know what I wanted to do with my free time. I had lost touch with what having a good time meant anymore.

When Diane and I started ImpactParents.com, our website asked, "What do you need today?" It's a question most of us don't consider often enough. Instead, we focus on the needs of those around us, without giving much thought to our own. So, I want to help you get clear for yourself what self-care really means for you. Brainstorm what kinds of things, large or small, make you feel good. What nourishes you? What puts fuel in your tank? What jazzes you? Maybe it's:

- making a date with your partner or friends;
- joining a softball team;
- getting your nails done;
- reading a good book;
- affirmations or one-minute meditations;
- pausing to take a breath or move your body each day;
- hiking;
- singing or listening to music (maybe really loudly);
- your kids' laughter;
- walking the dog;
- soaking in a tub;
- sunsets;

- a glass of wine or a cup of tea;
- practical jokes;
- painting;
- jigsaw puzzles; and/or
- guilty-pleasure movies;
- delicious dark chocolate.

It doesn't matter what's on the list, only that you start to create one for yourself. I'm not suggesting that you structure time to make any of this happen, yet. For now, just get to know yourself again. You can implement later.

If you're not sure where to begin, think about what you enjoyed before you had kids. What do you value that has been difficult to make a priority in recent years? One dad I worked with, for example, realized that he loved being involved at church and had lost that connection when he had kids. The entire family was impacted positively when he started going to church for himself.

For many of us, making a commitment to taking care of ourselves is a challenge. We may feel guilt or embarrassment, like it's a waste of time, or that we need to put every extra ounce of energy into our kids. Because they've got "issues" and need so much, it's easy to let ourselves slide—and most of us do.

> We have to learn to give without giving ourselves away.

We have to learn to give without giving ourselves away. When you know clearly what you want, it's easier to fit it in over time, in small pieces at first. It starts with clarity. Then giving yourself permission. Then eventually you'll start making time for yourself because it becomes natural. "Wanting" for yourself becomes a gift for your family.

When you ask yourself what you want or need today, I want you to be able to answer it. Start by answering the simple question: what feeds you?

Questions for Self-Discovery

- Why don't kids have a "just get it done" button?
- What are the biggest executive function challenges in your home?
- Which motivators are best for each member of your family?
- What catastrophic thoughts worry you?
- What's the connection between ownership and rewards?
- What's on your list to nourish your mind, body, or soul?

TAMMY'S STORY

Tammy had a rough few weeks. Her daughter's anxiety had begun to spike after a change in ADHD medication, and it seemed more upheaval was ahead. She choked up as she talked about her worries for her child's future and her challenges with managing her own fears so she doesn't overwhelm her daughter. "I never had a good role model for parenting," she explained. "If I didn't have you, I really wouldn't know what to say, or how to say it. I don't want my daughter to grow up thinking about herself the way I did. I don't want her to think that she's bad. But I don't want to coddle her, either. I want her to see how amazing she is, and how strong she can be, without her giving up or me giving in all the time. This is so much harder than I ever expected."

Bottom Line: "I never had a good role model for parenting. This is so much harder than I ever expected. How do I help her without doing too much for her?"

CHAPTER 8

"Everyone's So Tense All the Time"

It's Not What You Say, It's How You Say It

PART TWO

> "When there is no more blame or criticism in your eyes, when you are able to look at others with compassion, you see things very differently. You speak differently. The other person can sense you are truly seeing her and understanding her, and that already eases her pain significantly." —THICH NHAT HANH

Chaos and Disappointment

One of my best friends used to live next door, and our combined six kids flowed comfortably in and out of each other's homes. Our house had a constant swirl, an unmistakable energy that seemed to spill across every open surface and threshold. Our neurotypical friend's home reflected his relatively quiet and subdued energy. Everything was in its place, no clutter to be found. Recently he confessed that there was a limit to the time he could spend in our home. He loved us, but it was too chaotic. He needed to retreat and regroup.

And so it is. There are beautiful moments in our lives with complex kids. We live for those moments. But sometimes there's a surreal layer that makes it hard to keep a sense of humor as drama unfolds. We get overwhelmed by the chaos and heavily burdened by disappointment. Sometimes we bear the weight with guilt or shame. It's truly a madman's paradise.

Upheaval is a normal part of everyone's life. Starting a school year or ending it, changing jobs, or even finding a new babysitter are times when we expect life's transitions to be a bit more challenging. But when the basic events of daily life routinely throw things off balance, it's not usually the kind of change you post on social media.

Most of us have experienced some of these moments. We've

- sat, head in hands, feeling powerless because you hear someone you love "losing it" in another room.
- witnessed a child spend hours torturing themselves over what "should" be 10 minutes of schoolwork.
- unleashed, aware we're saying things we'll deeply regret.
- scripted a thousand things to say in our heads, only to remain silent, day after day, week after week.
- felt like we're walking on eggshells, afraid to trigger a storm.
- listened to a child scream or watched them unravel, feeling powerless and unable to soothe or calm them.
- stood by feeling helpless as a child is hitting walls, throwing punches, and wreaking havoc.
- watched a child self-sabotage or quit on themselves.

In complex families, simple, everyday transitions cause uncertainty, which creates chaos. It's a hallmark of our kids' challenges that they don't deal well with transitions, and it's difficult to embrace change with open arms when smooth-running systems are easily derailed.

> With complex kids, we may feel like we're living in chaos—on steroids.

And so, we often feel disappointed or resentful, like we're failing our kids, failing at parenting, teaching, or life. We don't want to go home after work, or to plan family outings or new class activities, because the mere thought of "togetherness" makes us want to run away. We hate to admit that all too often we don't like these kids very much, so we begin to stop liking ourselves instead.

Transition is a hallmark of educating a child, and chaos is (generally speaking) a key foundation of family life. But with complex kids, we may feel like we're living in chaos on steroids. The only constant in life is change, which can be a wondrous adventure or an ominous, threatening taskmaster. Because not knowing is a fundamental component of our worlds, it helps to embrace the chaos—to understand and expect it, even respect and befriend it.

Coach's Reframe: Create a Positive Tone of the Home

I asked a group of third-grade girls to take turns in front of the room asking the same question: "Would you take your backpack off the table please?" Before each turn, I called out an emotion to express: kind, angry, impatient, sweet, annoyed, hungry, supportive, loving, hateful, sarcastic. The girls loved the game, laughing a lot. The mothers in the back of the room heard themselves in their daughters' voices. They didn't always like what they heard.

ARE YOU SECRETLY CALLING YOUR CHILD AN IDIOT?

Communication is contextual, happening in words, tone, expression, and gesture. Our choices can be empowering:

- "Yes, and . . . " instead of "but" can disarm defense mode.
- "Could" instead of "should" offers authentic choice and control.
- "What do you think?" instead of "Why don't you . . . ?" empowers ownership and independence.

Sometimes we inadvertently sabotage communication. We think we're masking frustration, disappointment, fear, judgment, shame, or blame, but our kids hear the truth in our tone, or our words tell another story:

- "What were you thinking?" ("You're an idiot.")
- "What on Earth?" ("You can't do anything right.")
- "For the tenth time . . . " ("You have no respect.")
- "Are you sure?" ("I don't trust you.")
- "Have you done what I asked?" ("You slacker.")
- "Why didn't you?" ("You're doomed to fail.")

It's curious how we're cautious with those we don't know, polite when addressing authority ("yes, ma'am"), and considerate when speaking to strangers ("please, go ahead"). But to our loved ones we can be downright mean, without meaning to be. Whatever makes you most frustrated or concerned is subtly expressed in your tone.

To shift your thoughts to improve your communication, try this:

1. Think about your worst fears or concerns for your child. Say it out loud and try to identify the tone you're unwittingly expressing in your voice.

2. Ask your spouse or BFF what worry tends to sneak out in your tone. Narrow it down to the 1 to 3 most likely messages.

3. Get curious about what else is also true besides your fears. Consider new thoughts that might be more helpful.

BEYOND TONE OF VOICE, TONE OF THE HOME

Whether you call it searching for a silver lining or spin control, a positive mindset will guide you to create a tone in your home that improves family life.

While negativity is toxic and breeds more negativity, positivity can help make a difficult situation better. When you shift your perspective (and the words and tone to reflect it) from adversarial to cooperative, it paves the way to better outcomes.

Positivity isn't just about being nice. It's about interpreting a situation in such a way that improves the future. It's not that Anne Frank kept a diary that was so spectacular, it's that she kept a positive perspective even in the face of some of the worst atrocities known to humankind that gave her story its impact and longevity.

Sometimes the details of what homework didn't get turned in, what chore didn't get done, or who's standing up at dinner should take a back seat to helping your child feel confident, connected, and loved. Let some things slide in the interest of helping kids see their strengths and feel supported.

To be honest, you might look at your sloppy teen hiding behind earphones, drumming at the table, and think, "ungrateful freeloader" while you ask him to "pass the butter, please." You're human, and they're frustrating at times. The challenge is to manage your tone of voice until you can redirect your thoughts to something more constructive for everyone.

What's good for our kids is actually great for us (and our relationships). To create a positive tone in your home when it feels like every day you're sinking into quicksand, keep focused on yourself, your child, and your relationships with each other. Let your kids know that you'll be there for them, even when things don't go the way you want. Conversation by conversation, focus on communicating with a positive tone of voice; over time, that will lead you to influence the tone of your home, creating a foundation for success that will last a lifetime—your child's lifetime.

Strategy: Play to Their Strengths

When my eldest child fell in love with acting during a third-grade after-school Shakespeare class, I had never seen them thrive in quite that way, no matter what therapies, doctors, or medicines they tried. Acting class was a win and became a constant. I joke that it was cheaper than therapy, but truthfully, I saw them light up and sensed it was essential. In a twist I never would have anticipated, playing to their strength turned into a career that changed their life forever.

This applies to adults, as well. When I learned what I call the maxim of ADHD coaching—play to your strengths and outsource your challenges— it changed my life. As I began to play to my strengths, I hired a bookkeeper to manage the *administrivia* that was bogging me down. I found a business partner in Diane Dempster, who complemented my skills. I learned to ask for help and stopped trying to be everything to everyone. Playing to my strengths freed me up for personal and professional success.

In the world of complex kids, playing to your strengths—and leveraging them appropriately—is a fundamental tactic. Its value cannot be overestimated. The following excerpt from an interview with Dr. Stephen Hinshaw during the 2019 ADHD Parent's Palooza (see Chapter 3) offers an insight relevant to *all* kids:

"You've got a kid who is not a traditional learner. You've got a kid who is not the world's most organized person in terms of binders and backpacks and whatever, but who's more creative than others. Maybe you've got some of those traits yourself. Appreciate it!

". . . If you cut through what people have been studying about what makes kids tick, for many generations now, if you could do one single thing, it would be to find something your kid loves and is good at and give them every opportunity to practice it and express that. This is a thought experiment, because we live in a world where there's a lot of pressures, and kids need treatment, parents need treatment. But this is where strength-based approaches to resilience are really important.

"Maybe your kid doesn't get fabulous grades in school; but man are they musical, or artistic, or athletic. Or maybe they're not so good socially because it's just overwhelming for them; but you get them in an individual task or connections online, and there's ways for kids to connect with other people without some of the stresses of being in a group all the time. Families need to figure out what you're good at, and reinforce the heck out of that, and give opportunities, not just dwelling on the negative. If I could give one piece of advice, that would be it." He continued, "stamp collecting, or playing with bugs, or the nontraditional sport that they're really good at, or music. . . . Help your kid find that area that they really enjoy and are good at and let them thrive in it.

"Because in the long run, the building of legitimate self-esteem, and the building of self-confidence from doing . . . I mean that's what keeps all of us going. Find something that you're really good at, you really enjoy doing, and then if you can do that, a lot of other stuff ends up going along for the ride with that."

Your kids have challenges. Instead of allowing them to be defined by them, let them be defined by their strengths and gifts. Find what they love and let them dive into it. Don't take them out of art class if they love art, just for more math tutoring. Focus on those things that make them feel terrific about themselves, as they're the source of future success. Don't keep it a secret either. More than likely, your child is frustrated too, and a reminder of their successes will make you both feel fabulous!

Say No to Perfectionism

For most of my life, I avoided failure at all costs. I pursued only opportunities at which I could excel and avoided anything I didn't do well. Narrowing my options reinforced an unhealthy fear of failure, and I let fear of striking out prevent me from playing the game.

Focus on those things that make them feel terrific about themselves, as they're the source of future success.

And then, I was gifted with a child significantly challenged by the complexities of life and learning. Their path veered outside the lines, which turned out to be my greatest teacher (despite my initial reluctance to be its student).

For years, I railed against my child's differences and danced around the edges of their "issues," buying diagnoses and therapies, trying everything in my power to ensure that my smart kid would be successful. I was determined that their life would be "normal," which in some twisted way meant perfect. But I was on a fool's errand.

Early in their elementary years, I started to learn a powerful lesson: To be the best parent possible for them, I had to let go of other people's definitions of success and stop dragging them, kicking and screaming, to my definition of their success. It took years to come to terms with my own "failure" to raise a "perfect" child. By the time that child was 12, I became a perfectionist in recovery, though there were no 12 steps in my program. Instead every day, I made the effort to see failure as an excellent teacher (alongside success).

To recognize, embrace, and accept complex kids for the humans they are and let go of some ideal notion of who they should be, we must shed our out-dated notions of perfectionism that leave us all feeling broken and worthless. When kids feel that perfection is the only acceptable standard, they tend to respond in one of two ways:

- Anxiety takes over, driving every action and decision, robbing them of feeling a sense of satisfaction in any accomplishment.
- Nothing is ever good enough, so eventually they give up and stop trying. It still stings that I was part of creating this truth for my child: "Don't you see, Mom? If I don't do it, then I haven't done it wrong!"

A drive for excellence leads to self-improvement and achievement, and there's nothing wrong with that. You're reading this book to improve the dynamic in your relationships with your kids, right? The challenge is to keep that drive from becoming tyrannical, to allow some things in life to be good enough. Focus on progress, not perfection.

Diane taught me a strategy to keep perfectionist demons at bay: G.E.M.O., which stands for Good Enough Move On. We use it in our company all the time. When you're working on a project or guiding your kids to learn something, notice when something is good enough and it's time to move on. Maybe you don't need to refold those shirts, reload the dishwasher, or correct those spelling sentences. What if they're actually good enough?

> Focus on progress, not perfection.

If you tend to insist on perfection, what might help you focus on your child's strengths? I'm not asking you to abandon values of achievement, but notice when those values interfere with your relationships, sleeping peacefully, and

PART TWO

feeling calm or even happy. The distinction between excellence and perfectionism is a fine line that a lot of us dance around, and we want to do that consciously, noticing when it gets in the way and when it helps.

Perfectionism works against us and our kids. Managing our own perfectionism models acceptance and a more realistic approach to achievement. At the end of the day, a 90 is still an A. Ask yourself—is that good enough?

Say Yes to Radical Compassion

Years ago, facilitator Shannon Kelly guided me through a Bigger Game workshop (created by Rick Tamlyn). I was seeking clarity about my mission to create a global resource for parents of complex kids. I can still feel the choke in my voice as I responded to her question about my purpose: ". . . so that no child will ever grow up feeling the way I did."

Three scraps of paper pinned on my office wall have moved with me from one space to another. They remind me of how hard it is to be a complex child, and the powerful benefits of parenting with a coach approach. The first two quotes arrived shortly after I started coaching, when my preteen started to share what they were feeling because I was open to listening. These words struck me as sad and poignant:

"I don't mean to be so dysfunctional."

"The minute she started yelling at me, I put it out of my mind."

Another message, written on a cute little sticky note in their handwriting a few years later, after I started practicing radical compassion, fills me with hope:

"When life kicks you, let it kick you foreward [sic]. Be proud and unafraid to make mistakes. Be you."

When we're exasperated and exhausted, at the end of a long day or at the beginning of an overextended week, with too many commitments and too little time, it's hard to remember that our kids are suffering. We just want them to behave, or follow directions, or do what's expected of them, so we can do what's expected of us. We easily forget that what we see as a simple hurdle to overcome, they may experience as an insurmountable mountain. Complex kids are struggling.

> Strong relationships are at the core of helping children improve their behaviors.

My clients tell me that they say things to their kids that they regret. They're worried about their kids' self-esteem or concerned that their kids are apathetic and lazy. Driven to teach, guide, shape, and prepare kids for the big, bad world, they feel mandated to hold them accountable, applying just punishments and appropriate consequences—a signal to the world that they take their role seriously, are responsible adults, and are in control.

Parents try threats, idle warnings, and removal of privileges. We take away everything until there's nothing left to take away. It's hard to remember our kids aren't avoiding work just to be rude, difficult, or disrespectful. They don't have a mechanism to get themselves activated, organized, or self-regulated. And they find that embarrassing (and demoralizing). They certainly don't need us reminding them constantly, much less making them feel bad about it.

Your kids want to be seen, heard, and understood. They want their perspective and experience to matter. They want to know that you're on their team. That's how you will successfully guide them to independence.

Shame and blame will not help your child perform better. It damages your relationships, reducing your child's ability to trust you, reinforcing negative self-images, and making it harder for kids to get their stuff done. If they feel like you don't really understand what it's like for them, why should they bother trying?

I'm not saying that all you need is love and connection, but strong relationships are at the core of helping children improve their behaviors. Radical compassion gives you permission to feel for your kids' experience, an access point to empower them to see what's possible for themselves, instead of only focusing on what they feel is "broken."

Self-Talk: Make It Okay to Make Mistakes (and Stop the Lying)

Sarah Blakely, founder of Spanx, attributes her father's celebration of mistakes as a key factor to her success. Despite her lack of experience, it never occurred to her that she couldn't do it. Similarly, we wouldn't have potato chips, the Slinky, Scotch Guard, the pacemaker, fireworks, Post-it notes, or chocolate chip cookies without mistakes. Alexander Fleming forgot to clean his petri dishes in the lab before he closed the windows and left for vacation. He came back to a moldy mess—and changed the course of medical history with the discovery of penicillin.

Even though mistakes are a fundamental component of human success, we tend to freak out when we or our kids make them. And when kids feel wrong all the time, their self-esteem diminishes and they cover up, stop trying, or create ways to be right. On coaching calls, Diane and I frequently hear:

- "My son said he'd done his homework, but he hadn't."
- "He lied to me."
- "She looked me in the eye and lied about it."
- "I caught them in another lie."

Here's the truth: Kids lie. All the time. Even the really earnest, rule-following kids. Lying is exaggerated with complex kids—not because they're less honest, but because self-preservation leads to them to deny and defend themselves so that they don't feel that they are always wrong. I call it "defensive dishonesty." And we parents are partially to blame:

- We constantly correct kids, from little redirections to big lectures, exhausting everyone.
- Kids are literal and unsure when lies are okay. We tell them "Say you're sorry" when they aren't, or "Mom's not home" to avoid a phone call. Because kids intend to do their homework, can't they say it's already done?
- We're determined to catch them in a lie for their own good.

But you can create an environment that makes it okay to make mistakes by accepting that it's "normal" for a complex child to be physically or mentally overactive, impulsive, or whatever. You can take the shame, blame, annoyance, and embarrassment out of corrections and redirections. Make mistakes as matter-of-fact as possible. Model positive reactions ("Whoops, I broke the kitchen faucet"), teach that mistakes are learning experiences ("Next time, I'll read the instruction manual"), and take the pressure off of everyone to always have to "get it right."

> Make mistakes as matter-of-fact as possible.

To make it okay to make mistakes, try to

- Limit corrections and save redirections for what's important.
- Keep a sense of humor when you make corrections.
- Have "no correction" time with your kids (don't tell them; just don't correct anything that's not dangerous).
- Laugh at life's silly mistakes.
- Be open to constructive criticism and suggestions.

- Make mistakes matter-of-fact.
- Apply a scientific approach to what works and what doesn't.
- Verbalize mistakes (without making yourself wrong for them).

"Isn't it cute that you think you're going to remember?" I ask my child with working memory challenges, followed by "What are you going to do to help yourself remember?" That same kid is likely to say playfully, "I don't know what you mean, Mom, of course I didn't leave my dirty dishes in the family room; what would you expect of me?" while he's belatedly bringing the dishes to the kitchen. Sure, I could yell at him for not doing it originally. Or I could thank him for taking care of it with good humor, keeping a positive tone in our home, and reinforcing our connected relationship.

Mistakes are going to happen—more in our homes than others—and our reaction to them really matters. Maybe you don't need to pick your mistakes out of the trash like Sir Fleming, but you can hold them lightly and remove the stigma for everyone. We are, as my eldest child likes to say, perfectly imperfect.

Questions for Self-Discovery

- What's disappointing for you?
- How do you create a positive tone in your home?
- What are your child's strengths?
- When does perfectionism have a hold on you?
- Where do you feel compassion for your child?
- How do you handle making mistakes?

ELIJAH'S STORY

Elijah explained: My wife has a high-powered job. I'm the primary caretaker and work part time. I love it. The kids really respond to me, but things are not nearly as peaceful when she's around. I want her to enjoy spending time with the family, and I want the kids to like being with their mum. But my wife doesn't understand their issues well, and she doesn't have patience or flexibility. Even though the kids are doing the best they can and just need a little extra support, she thinks they're not trying and that I'm babying them too much. I don't know how to help her see that there's so much more than grades and following directions. Truly, our kids are so amazing—I want to help her relax and enjoy our family instead of creating so much friction in the home.

Bottom Line: The kids are well-behaved with one parent, but it's stressful when both parents are around. Unrealistic expectations are keeping one parent from enjoying a great relationship with the kids.

CHAPTER 9

"I Don't Know What's Realistic"

Set Appropriate Expectations and Consequences

"But nonjudgmentally recognizing and embracing this great suffering is not at all the same thing as giving in to it." —THICH NHAT HANH

Unreasonable Expectations and Developmental Delays

"Exorbitant expectations are a set-up, and when they don't work out, they boomerang back to disillusion you. Better to tackle big and complex problems realistically and with humility." —Paul Bianchi, Headmaster, Paideia School

Imagine your child breaks their wrist and gets a cast that goes from hand to elbow, just as their class is learning cursive writing. They watch the lessons on cursive, even try it with their nondominant hand. But they never get a chance to really learn the cursive. By the next school year, there's no cast, and the teacher expects that they "should" know cursive (which they do in theory, but not in practice).

This scenario plays out repeatedly with complex kids, who tend to be behaviorally, socially, and/or emotionally immature, despite potentially being cognitively advanced. In essence, deficits in executive function reflect about a 30% developmental delay in some aspects of their brain development—though not all—such that complex kids are typically behind their same-age peers in some areas by about 3 to 5 years.

These inconsistencies are extremely confusing for adults. Complex kids can:

- have mature conversations or make compelling arguments, while being unable to clean their room, remember to take out the trash, or turn in homework.
- have great friends, but seem unable to manage their anger or frustration with their family.
- do well in school, but lag behind socially.
- be confident socially but unable to organize themselves and do school.
- perform well one week but not the next, with no apparent cause for the erratic behavior.

Despite understanding this intellectually, when we evaluate kids' behaviors in comparison to their neurotypical peers, we're not making a fair comparison. We're disappointed when they don't perform on par with their peers. We say things like, "but he's 8 years old, he should know better than to . . . " or "she's 12, shouldn't she be able to . . . ?"

- We get stuck on how something "should" be, how a child "should" behave, or how something "should" look to the outside world. We expect our kids to behave like older siblings or our friends' kids.
- We worry about the implications of "settling for less" or "lowering our standards." They are bright with extraordinary potential. We set expectations high so they don't waste that potential.
- We need them to be okay for us to feel calm and in control, as Hal Runkel explains in *ScreamFree Parenting*. When they're feeling sad, we need them to be happy; when they're falling behind in school, we need them to be organized; when they're emotionally sensitive, we need them to toughen up.

As parents, we're committed to helping kids reach their full potential, so I'm not arguing for removing expectations, or even lowering them. "You can't parent or teach without expectations. Expectations are how you communicate your experience, wisdom, and values," Ross Greene said during his 2019 International Conference on ADHD keynote. But "pushing a kid to meet an expectation you know he can't meet" based on age, without taking developmental delays into account, generally leads to unwanted behaviors.

Coach's Reframe: Meet Them Where They Are and Raise the Bar from There

My client's son was a very bright teen who was failing two classes, getting Bs and Cs in two more, and getting an A in honors history. Classic. He loved his history teacher and was bored in his other classes. But summer school was on the horizon if he didn't turn those two Fs around. He was intellectually capable of getting straight As, but he hadn't learned to master his motivation, so he was struggling just to pass.

If his mom had delivered ultimatums, he would have likely spent the summer in school. Instead, she met her son where he was. She held her tongue about her disappointment, resisting the temptation to tell him he needed to get his act together, which he already knew. She talked with him about what he wanted to do for the summer, what it would take to pass the classes, and if he wanted that. They put together a plan, including check-ins and accountability, to meet his goal of having a summer break.

At first, this mom was apoplectic. But she kept her own fears and emotions out of the conversation, helping him think through what it would take to raise his grades in two classes. She stayed calm and present with his current circumstance, and she managed her own catastrophizing (see Chapter 7). Her calm approach helped him raise the bar and avoid summer school.

It's a catch-22, really. Our kids struggle with challenges invisible to the naked eye, and we often set expectations based on wishful thinking. But when we set the bar too high for them, expecting them to perform and hit typical milestones that they're not ready for, it's like telling them to grow taller. Complex kids need:

- to believe that they're capable;
- permission to take extra time in getting there;
- to learn to overcome obstacles without embarrassment or shame; and
- support to understand the process.

To meet them where they are, we must be matter of fact, inviting them to take the next step forward. As one coaching group mom explained, "[I must] commit to look at my own behavior to make sure that I'm setting appropriate boundaries for my child."

The greatest gift you can give yourself, and any complex child, is to acknowledge and accept the challenges they're facing and encourage them to move forward from exactly where they are.

You wouldn't ask a nearsighted kid to sit in the back of the room and squint to read from the board. You wouldn't tell them to try harder or argue that their friends can see, so they should be able to as well. Instead, you'd provide an accommodation for the nearsightedness so that the student could be successful, and then encourage them to use that accommodation without embarrassment. Maybe you'd move them to the front of the room so they can see the board or get them glasses. If they resisted, you'd offer encouragement, helping them see the value for them in wearing glasses.

One of our certified Sanity School® trainers is a fourth-grade teacher-of-the-year who uses the coach approach in her classroom. When she noticed the bar was set too high for one student, she reduced the expectations, and he started to perform. When the bar was too high, he wasn't willing to try.

> Positivity is not enough. Complex kids need us to shift *our* expectations. It's fundamental to *their* success.

Setting appropriate expectations—as teachers, parents, and even students—starts with reframing mindset. We want to focus on incremental growth. Progress not perfection. Keep it manageable and realistic. And, most of all, empower kids by showing them that wherever they are is just fine.

As I used to say to my own kids quite frequently, "Patience, young grasshopper. You're going to be an amazing adult, we just gotta get you there."

Strategy: Shift Expectations with the 3–5 Challenge

At 17, my eldest overheard me in the kitchen explaining the 3- to 5-year delay to a neighbor. They came into the kitchen and said, "Wait, Mom, do you mean I'm not really an immature 17-year-old? I'm really a mature 12-year-old?" I laughed, "Well, sort of, yes." "Cool," they replied. "I can be with that." And they have.

In fact, it was liberating for them. It was always confusing that they were so mature in some areas and frighteningly immature in others. Shifting expectations leveled the playing field, helping them continue to move forward with less shame, confident they would eventually catch up.

Although positivity is a common thread that runs through every parenting paradigm I've ever studied, and it's essential to everything in this book, I want to be clear: Positivity is not enough. Complex kids need us to shift *our* expectations. It's fundamental to *their* success.

TAKE THE 3-5 CHALLENGE

When you're frustrated that your child is not performing a task how you think they should, or you find yourself thinking, "Why can't they just," here's how to modify your expectations.

1. **Ask yourself, "What do I expect in this scenario?"** Think clearly and specifically.

2. **Subtract 3 to 5 years from the child's age.** (If it's early morning or after 5 pm, subtract two more.) Ask yourself, "What age does this child seem like to me in terms of this task?" Is she 9 going on 10, or more like 9 going on 6?

3. **Ask yourself, "Would it be reasonable to expect a child 3 to 5 years younger to complete this task independently?"** What might be a more realistic expectation?

When you think about a seventh-grader as a fourth-grader, developmentally, what do you notice? Are you still surprised they're failing to meet expectations? You may observe several factors that indicate a 3- to 5-year delay, such as:

They aren't ready to do the task independently. During those times when they are straining, they need extra scaffolding and support. Children with working memory challenges, for example, often need an external structure to aid in remembering.

They don't quite know what to do. When a particular skill was taught, they may not have been available to learn it. Like the child with the broken arm who never learned cursive, they may need to be taught again, now that they're ready.

They can do it sometimes, but not consistently. Complex kids are wired to be erratic, so inconsistent performance is reasonable to

NATURAL CONSEQUENCES AT AGE 16

This story demonstrates how transferring ownership takes time (see Chapter 4). "I've got it, Mom," he said, packing for a lengthy summer program, resisting help with time or organization. He packed himself. On the first night, he texted:

"I forgot sheets and a pillow."

"Bummer man." (Confession: Privately, I laughed out loud.)

"I guess you want me to send something?" (Letting him ask for our help.)

"Yes please. sheets and a pillow, por favor" (No reply— let him squirm a bit.)

A few hours later: "and some shower towels" Pause. "and my water bottle leaks."

My husband replied: "Guess we need to send a bottle too?" (Again, letting him ask for help.)

"Yes please. please and thank you." Pause. "I borrowed sheets. using a sweatshirt as a pillow and I don't have towels." (Natural consequence + asking for help with gratitude!)

The next morning, I texted. "Will do our best but will likely take several days. Oh, do you need a blanket?"

"Yes, I need a blanket. not urgent, but it would be nice."

My husband adds, "$23 to get there Tuesday. $185 to get there Monday. Do you want to pay $185?"

"Nope. Thank you."

Eleven hours later, the package already on its way, the final text arrived:

"Is it too late to ask for a laundry bag?"

"Already sent it :-). Good night kid."

Natural consequences helped my son learn from mistakes in a way that lecturing him never could, keeping us on the same team. It cost him $23, he asked for help many times, and he learned to appreciate us and his pillow. He didn't blame us, and was grateful. I never said, "I told you so." The hardest part was not teasing him mercilessly.

That satisfaction came two years later, procrastinating while packing for college. "I've got it, Mom." He was adamant he was on top of things, claiming to be the best packer in the family. We sparred jokingly for a week. At the right moment, I read him the text thread above. He conceded to a friend, "She got me. And she even has evidence to prove it." The sheets, towels, and blankets made it that time.

expect. To pay attention, for example, many aspects of executive function are required, influenced by factors such as sufficient sleep, social connections, or whether they find the subject interesting.

They may be inconsistent across areas of performance. A 12-year-old motivated by soccer may be organized in that realm, but still unable to apply those skills to perform in school.

They may slide back in one area when they're working on growth in another. When kids take on new activities, roles (like a lead in a school musical or president of a club), or jobs (work outside of school), they experience exponential growth. But it can compromise their schoolwork. Even the most independent students may need extra support when circumstances change, such as during exams.

When a teacher started using this strategy after taking Sanity School for Teachers, she noticed significant changes in her classroom. She was resistant at first, not wanting to see her kindergarten students as 3-year-olds. But as she shifted her expectations, it allowed her to successfully integrate all students in a classroom of five- and six year olds.

In a recent training for professionals becoming certified to teach our Sanity School course to parents or teachers in local communities, Katie summed it up best: "understanding that 3- to 5-year delay is a game-changer."

Say No to Punishment Disguised as Consequences

"You're grounded for a year!"

We've all thought it. Some of us have said it. Most of us regret it.

If you've ever created a consequence that's more of a punishment for you than it is for your kids, or if you've threatened an unrealistic punishment, you're not alone. Sometimes we get so frustrated, a punishment slips out before we can stop ourselves. It's defeating for our kids and demoralizing for us. Sometimes it turns into a punishment disguised as consequences:

- "If you don't clean your room, you'll lose your favorite game."
- "If you don't get to the bus on time, you'll lose your sleepover."
- "If you talk to me like that again, you'll lose the computer for the rest of the term."

PART TWO

In the old days, parents were taught to respond to bad behaviors with punishments; now we're taught to use consequences, ideally natural consequences. What's the difference? Punishment is a punitive measure intended to cause pain or discomfort in order to discourage future behaviors. Think: washing a child's mouth out with soap so they won't use foul language. Consequences are intended to link outcomes with learning experiences in order to change future behaviors. Think: expecting a child to pay for a broken window so they won't throw balls in the house in the future. Natural consequences are outcomes that are not necessarily imposed by a parent but happen naturally as a result of a mistake or problem. Think: a failed test may remind a child to study more in the future.

> It's more important to help them learn from their mistakes than any consequence you feel the need to impose.

When complex kids do something "wrong," we feel compelled to respond so they'll learn from their mistake. Unfortunately, our consequence is often a punishment in disguise. It's not particularly fair to randomly impose threats, use guilt, issue idle warnings, and take things away. How can kids avoid the punishment if they don't know it's coming?

Diane and I often get calls from parents who say, "I just don't know what to do anymore. There's nothing left for me to take away, and my child doesn't seem to care at all!" When kids are struggling to get their brains to respond the way they know they *should*, constant disapproval and retroactive consequences add insult to injury; they lead to either giving up or rebellion.

Instead, it's more important to help them learn from their mistakes than any consequence you feel the need to impose.

Incentives (helping kids identify motivation to improve their behaviors) and natural consequences can work magic when used appropriately, especially when you keep it light and keep your sense of humor. When realistic expectations are set in advance, clearly communicated and agreed upon, then appropriate consequences can be established—and help our kids learn to self-manage. When your kid knows what to expect and you can "let the system be the bad guy," a consequence does the teaching while you stay on your kids' team with compassion.

Say Yes to Championing and Seeing Possibilities (Foster Resilience)

"In 1955, researchers Emmy Werner (University of California, Davis) and Ruth Smith (licensed psychologist, Kauai) began a longitudinal study that followed all of the children born on the island of Kauai during that year." Many of the students were raised in difficult circumstances and developed significant problems by age 10. But about one-third of those challenged children did very well in life.

Werner and Smith called them "vulnerable, but invincible." The kids who "showed the most resiliency were those who had access to buffering elements known as 'protective factors,'" including emotional support in and outside of the family. It turned out, when kids had one adult who believed in them, one adult they could turn to in times of strife, it made a significant difference in their outcomes.

Our kids, more than most, need us to see what's possible for them, and help them see it for themselves. They get so many messages from the world that tell them they're not enough—not good enough, smart enough, fast enough, organized enough, calm enough. I recently said to a friend whose child suffers from anxiety, "Your job is not to protect them from it. Your job is to help them through it."

We do that with strategies, tactics, and so many things we're covering in this book. And we also do that by holding a vision for them until they're able to hold it for themselves. That's how we cultivate their ability to see themselves as resilient, to believe that they'll be able to achieve whatever vision they have for themselves.

Our kids are at risk of vulnerability, but we can help them see themselves as invincible. I don't mean "I don't need to wear a seatbelt" invincibility; more like "life is hard but people believe in me and I can do this" invincibility. We can have an enormous impact simply by believing in our kids, seeing what's possible for them, and inviting them to believe in themselves. We can guide them to discover and embrace their own resilience.

Our kids notice when we highlight what's broken or what could go wrong, even when we don't realize we're doing it. When we get upset and demand better performance after a poor report card, for example, we want to make sure we're sending the message that we believe they can do better, not that we're afraid they can't. With that, they're more likely to believe in themselves.

PART TWO

I wrote once that the 10 most important words a parent could say to their child were "I believe in you. I know you can do it!" It's positive, affirming, and empowering. But my friend Jerome Schultz, PhD, author of *Nowhere to Hide*, advised me to avoid adding additional pressure. Now I encourage parents to say something like, "I believe you can do it. I know you might not be sure, yourself. That's okay. For now, trust that I see what you can do, and I'll hold that belief for you until you're ready to take it on for yourself."

Shifting expectations is not to be confused with settling for "less" or "low-ering" your expectations. The goal here is to set realistic expectations in the short term, and hold a powerful vision of who our kids can be and what they can achieve in the long term.

Self-Talk: Assume Best Intentions (A.B.I.)

I remember Don Knotts drawing on a courtroom chalkboard during an epi-sode of *Mayberry RFD*: ASS-U-ME. "When you assume," he said, "You make an ass out of you and me." Who says there's nothing to learn from television?

Making assumptions can trigger a cycle of miscommunication that can spiral out of control and interfere with relationships. Say your child has been in trouble at school because she's forgotten her homework. You find out only because her teacher emails you. "But, Mom, I didn't want you to get mad." (Which you are, because she didn't tell you.) She made an assumption about your response that prevented open communication.

It's not realistic to expect any of us to stop making assumptions. But because we choose interpretations to manage the ups and downs of life, we *can* choose to make helpful assumptions.

In coaching we say, "it's all made up." We understand that people are going to make assumptions, because that's how brains work. Everything is filtered through perception, and we frequently take action based on what we assume about a situation, even when we don't know for sure. Our kids do it all the time too. So, we might as well make our assumptions work for us by reframing how we think about them.

Diane taught me a tool that has become a gold standard tactic for every parents' toolbox. We call it A.B.I., Assume Best Intention. If you go to the homes of our clients, you may see "ABI" on sticky notes peppered around the house. It's a subtle reminder of the power of making up assumptions that work for you. As an added bonus, kids have no idea what it means.

A.B.I. reminds you to look for what's positive and possible. Start with the idea that your kids could be doing their best, or at least that they want to do their best. When your kids aren't following directions, instead of jumping to the conclusion that they're being disrespectful or disobedient, you could assume that your child is trying hard and wants to do their best. Your interpretation, over time, actually helps your child do better.

It can be so difficult for your kids to know what they "should" be able to do, to see their friends and siblings doing it, and not be able to do it themselves. It's incredibly frustrating for them. When you consider what it must be like for them to feel like they're constantly disappointing you, trying hard without success, you'll find a compassion you may not have had before.

With A.B.I., you're less likely to jump on little mistakes and more likely to acknowledge when things are harder than they seem like they should be. It goes a long way to avoiding major upsets too, because often our kids' meltdowns come from feeling misunderstood. It also gives you a different perspective to approach problem solving.

So, when your child isn't listening or following directions, or is so easily distracted that you want to pull your hair out, remind yourself that it's likely not a case of "willful disobedience." As you approach frustrating situations, remind yourself that your child is trying their best—and watch as it lightens the load and reduces the stress for everyone.

You might try to apply ABI to yourself, as well. At the 2019 Conference on ADHD, Dr. Ross Greene, known for his maxim "Kids do well if they can," added, "By the way, adults do well if they can too."

Questions for Self-Discovery

- How is your child delayed developmentally?
- Where will you start meeting them where they are?
- What did you learn by taking the 3–5 challenge?
- Are you punishing or establishing useful consequences?
- What's your vision for your child's future?
- What unhelpful assumptions do you tend to make?

PART TWO

HANNAH'S STORY

Hannah's mother abandoned her when she was 8, and her marine father ran a tight ship, micromanaging every step. With her first tastes of freedom, she was out of control. After eight years in college, a failed early marriage, and substance abuse, Hannah wanted things to be different for her son Miles. By his junior year, though, her micromanagement caused their relationship to fray at the seams. By senior year, Hannah started getting coaching so she could let go of her need to control. When Miles was at risk of not graduating, I asked, "What's the worst thing that could happen?" Hannah describes an "incredible peace" when she realized she accepted where he was. Hannah supported him in figuring out what to do and he did manage to graduate, though didn't go immediately to college because he hadn't applied on time. Hannah supported him without judgment and actually enjoyed the semester Miles worked and saved money as he watched his friends go off to college. Without making excuses, he said, "You know, Mom, maybe I should have applied sooner."

Bottom Line: The tighter you hold on, the less reason they have to take responsibility for themselves. You have to loosen the reins to transfer control.

CHAPTER 10

"I Need a Strategy for . . ."

Creating Effective Systems and Structures That Actually Work

"We ourselves need help. The other person also needs help.
Nobody needs punishment." —THICH NHAT HANH

Missing the Forest for the Trees: Starting with Solutions

"I want strategies."

"How do I get my child to do his homework?"

"I just want some peace."

"I'm yelling more than I'd like."

"My kid won't turn in her homework."

"The alarm clock doesn't help."

"They ignore me."

"They're so rude."

"She's freaking out all the time."

"I'm walking on eggshells."

"It's like he's hijacked the whole house."

"I don't want to go home."

It's hard to keep ourselves calm and our head (relatively) clear when deep inside we want to scream, "Stop, let me off!" After thousands of conversations, I've learned that all parents of complex kids, whether newbies or veterans, want the same two things: solutions and peace. They generally assume that the former will lead to the latter; actually, it's the other way around.

We humans love answers. We love systems, processes, and solutions. We love a good fix for an aggravating problem. But we're impatient and we don't always want to spend the time or effort needed to solve a problem thoughtfully. Instead we apply solutions without clarifying the problem in the first place. We throw spaghetti at the wall to see what sticks.

Unfortunately starting with solutions (strategies, systems, and structures) comes at a cost: kids don't learn to solve problems for themselves. When we give kids solutions that we think they should try or that others have used, they miss the chance to figure out what works for them. We might be giving them a nice fish dinner, but we're not teaching them to fish, much less how to plan a fishing trip.

When we give kids planners to use in school, buy unusual alarm clocks for home, or use graphic organizers to manage time, we often fail to achieve the desired results. It's not because systems and structures are not essential— they are. I'd have had a difficult time writing this book without calendars, computers, and sticky notes. But the goal of any solution is not to use the system or structure; it's to achieve a desired outcome.

STRATEGIES, SYSTEMS, AND STRUCTURES (OH MY!)

Although most people use the terms strategies, systems, and structures interchangeably, I think it's helpful to clarify them.

> **Strategies:** Ways to approach making improvements. A **strategy** to help a child get started on homework after school might be to activate the brain.

> **Systems:** The processes or routines we put into place to help us get things done. High-protein snacks or physical activity are **systems** for the strategy of activating the brain.

> **Structures:** The components of systems and routines. Bringing a protein snack in carpool or going straight to the playground from the bus are different **structures** a parent might use to implement a system for the strategy of activating the brain.

For example, to help a child perform better in the classroom, the team might choose a **strategy** of helping them stop interrupting during class. To provide incentives for the child to change their behavior, a reward **system** is chosen. Stars or points are **structures** used by the teacher to reinforce the child's positive behavior.

Chronic conditions actually require behavioral change, which is all about process. Strategies, systems, and structures are valuable tools for helping the brain compensate for challenges with executive function; but we must always remember that they are not the goal. They are tools to aid us in reaching a much broader and more important goal: helping kids learn self-management and self-regulation. You cannot accomplish long-term personal success with a system; instead, it requires a *process* of problem solving.

Coach's Reframe: Think Problem Solving, Not Fixing

For many years I was just trying to get through each day. I bounced pinball-style from solution to solution, looking for answers. We tried every traditional therapy known to medicine and a bunch of alternative approaches as well. Some helped, others didn't.

I was attracted to every shiny promise that "this" would fix everything, looking for a single solution that would make all our problems go away. With each new therapy or program, I (secretly) hoped I'd found a magic bullet. It makes me a little queasy to reflect on the thousands of dollars we spent.

I wasn't approaching things systematically as part of a bigger plan; and frankly, I wasn't looking for incremental improvement. I didn't understand that my kids' challenges fundamentally called for long-term behavior management. I just wanted a quick fix.

We want our kids to be able to grow into capable, independent adults. To be able to set goals and work hard to achieve them, navigating life's challenges and overcoming obstacles. We want them to engage in their lives, build healthy relationships, embark on fulfilling careers, and ultimately, support themselves as adults, so they don't end up living in our basements in twenty years or worse!

To achieve this long-term goal, we must avoid the temptation of magical thinking that happens when we go for a quick fix. Instead, we must do for ourselves what our kids need to learn: embrace the complicated, slow process of problem solving.

That doesn't mean you shouldn't try new things or put new systems into place. But do it thoughtfully. Become mindful of the process you use to introduce new "solutions." Let the Impact Model guide you to understand what you're trying to change and what's contributing to those behaviors. Then plan strategically: activate the brain (see Chapter 7), be positive (see Chapter 8), shift expectations (see Chapter 9), and make systems and structures work.

Before I discovered the coach approach, I believed I could "fix" my kids' problems. I thought we could eliminate them with a medicine, therapy, special school program, or social skills class. It wasn't until I learned the value of focusing on the process of problem solving that I stopped trying to rescue them from their challenges. Taking on a growth mindset was the path to lasting change.

> Embrace the complicated, slow process of problem solving.

Stephen Covey says to start with the end in mind, but that does not mean he's an advocate of quick fixes. He is talking about setting a vision of what you want to achieve, identifying the change you want to see, so that you can discover an effective process that leads to change.

Our kids need to learn constructive problem-solving skills, appropriate to where they are developmentally. And so do we. Instead of telling them "you've got to pass your classes to avoid summer school" or "you've got to get straight As to use the car," we must guide them through figuring out *how* to pass or do well in their classes. And that includes helping them find their motivation— getting clear on what's in it for them.

In the rest of this chapter, I'll focus on some key components to make systems and structures work effectively, holding the mindset that we are not trying to fix anything; rather, our goal is to improve one challenge at a time, one process at a time.

Strategy: Failing Forward (with Three Magic Questions)

"If you want to get better at anything, you need to experiment with an open mind, to try and fail, to willingly accept and learn from any outcome." —Peter Bregman, "Stop Focusing on Your Performance," *Harvard Business Review*

Here's something most of us hate: failure is a fundamental part of learning. We don't learn to talk without babbling or walk without stumbling. Scientific discovery relies on learning from failures, identifying what doesn't work without judgment so we can discover what does work. Failure is responsible for chocolate chip cookies, so it can't be all bad! (See Chapter 9) But still, most of us resist it with every fiber of our being.

It's reasonable to expect our kids to fail, falter, and make mistakes while learning to succeed, but *they* don't see it that way. They've been conditioned to want simple fixes, as you have; and they're often not exactly the most patient people. They're easily embarrassed and want to be seen as capable, by you and by themselves. Failure is the last thing they want to experience. They want to avoid mistakes at all costs.

Thus, teaching them to handle failure is an essential component of raising complex kids. It's difficult both because they tend to hate failure and because they don't learn from mistakes very efficiently. Because kids don't process mistakes while they're happening or they resist redirection out of shame, they often don't learn to avoid making the same mistakes again.

Patience with the process of problem solving and learning from mistakes can be overwhelming, frustrating, or scary for kids, and for us. As parents, we want to rescue them, limiting their frustration and disappointment in themselves.

But preventing them from experiencing failure reinforces their tendency to see themselves as stupid or flawed when they do make mistakes. Instead, we want to be on their team when they falter, brushing off the dust without judgment, so they can learn from the experience and discover how resilient they are.

Mistakes are human. It's up to us to give kids permission to be human with grace, and teach them to fail forward.

The strategy of failing forward is a magic process for learning from mistakes without shame or embarrassment. From the sublime to the ridiculous, in professional and personal settings, it works wonders. When a test score isn't great or a recipe kinda flops, try asking the three questions on page 142.

We want to set kids up for success whenever possible, collaborating with them as they learn to navigate life. Embrace a "practice makes perfect" mindset, paying attention to circumstances around mistakes only to learn from them. Avoid feeding feelings of inadequacy that lead kids to shut down. Help them learn from mistakes and establish new behaviors by failing forward, activating their brains to become more alert and aware in subsequent situations.

The bottom line here is to teach your kids, "Let every mistake be a new one." That will help them become less likely to repeat the same types of mistake and less likely to beat themselves up for making the first one. It's a great message for kids to hear—and not a bad one for us either.

THREE MAGIC QUESTIONS TO FAIL FORWARD

1. What worked? The essence of learning from mistakes is to start with the positive. This sets a tone of optimism and possibility and prevents people from going on the defensive.

2. What didn't work? After exploring the positive, discover other relevant details. Pay attention to what there is to learn from the mistake, matter-of-factly. Visit but don't dwell there.

3. What will you do differently? Start planning for the next attempt.

Say No to Results

At an Atlanta Women's Foundation annual luncheon, I heard Jane Pauley speak about her life with bipolar disorder. Her presentation was quietly intense, at times raw and poignant, and ultimately uplifting. She explained, "nobody gets through life without something." We all have our challenges.

With episodic diseases, things get better for a time, and then they rear their ugly head again. The key to any chronic condition, she explained, is management. Conscious, vigilant, lifelong management. And so it is for complex kids.

The ends justify the means. Outcomes measurement. Getting to the finish line. Many of us live in an end-goal kind of a culture. We want our kids to be successful, which we evaluate in terms of results. Our "solution-oriented" mindset focuses on where they're going, not how they get there.

We ask: did they get an A on a test? Did they score a goal in the game? Did they get an internship, or a job, or a license, or into a school? The measurement is the indicator of success: the prize, the pot of gold.

But reaching the goal doesn't always help kids learn to be successful in life. We can enable them to get an A or manage logistics so they get their license; but if they don't understand or can't replicate what it takes to achieve the result, are they actually learning from the experience?

PROCESS OVER OUTCOME

Have you heard about the snow-plow parent? That's the parent who removes all the obstacles in front of a child so they can move forward unobstructed. But what happens when we clear the path for our kids without helping them see the obstacles and learn to move around them? Is that really success?

For our kids to learn to manage the details of their lives and work, the processes of life *really* matter. It's like getting partial credit on a complicated math problem. How you solve the problem is as important as getting the right answer. Instead of holding your kids accountable to an outcome, help them see the process it takes to get there. Reward incremental steps, depending on age and ability.

- Instead of focusing on completing homework, reward them for staying on task for 10 to 20 minutes.
- Instead of punishing outbursts, reward their progress in managing emotions using self-calming strategies.
- Instead of telling them to take a time-out, reward them for choosing a technique to calm down when they're upset.
- Instead of criticizing a paper written at the last minute, acknowledge them for doing an outline in advance.
- Instead of bringing home a job application for them, give them kudos for talking to a manager and asking for one.
- Instead of emailing your child's teacher without including them in the conversation, celebrate them for talking to the teacher after school.

Help schools see the importance of this, too:

- Make sure reward systems in the classroom are focused on process, not just results.
- Help teachers understand that learning *how* may be more important than whether the child masters this week's spelling words or completes a five-page report.
- Focus on individual steps (one paragraph, instead of one page), allowing the child to experience incremental successes.

When we evaluate success only in terms of end results, we neglect the important role that conscious management plays in creating a sustainable life.

PART TWO

We want our kids to learn *how* to get the results they want in life. Whenever you start using a new system, focus your accountability on using the system rather than on the end result. Routines takes time, so reward the incremental steps along the way.

Say Yes to Keeping It Simple and Flexible

Try your best to be honest here. Do you . . .

- give long lectures . . . but your kids rarely process a word?
- put detailed systems into place . . . and then get aggravated when they don't work?
- try to tackle too many things at once . . . until everyone feels overwhelmed?
- demand consistency . . . and miss opportunities for compassionate learning?

My friend, you're not alone. On tough days, we nag, cajole, and bargain. We do anything to feel like we're making progress. But sometimes, we make things more complicated than necessary, for ourselves and for them.

Two of my failed attempts at using behavior charts in my kids' early years were outrageously off the mark:

- One listed every task my kids needed to do from morning to night (see Chapter 5). Capturing the detail was helpful for me. My mistake was showing it to my kids, much less expecting them to do it all independently.
- Another was a set of unbelievably unrealistic expectations—enormous goals, such as "make mornings better" and "be respectful." (see Good Behavior Chart on page 145) I thought it was simpler, but it wasn't. Some days it was hard enough to find my keys. How was I going to remember to check off a dozen daily items on a list? And how were my kids supposed to know if they made mornings better?

To be implemented easily, effective solutions are a lot like a bridge. They've got a clear job to do, and you want to keep them simple and flexible so that using them doesn't become one more thing we fail at each day.

Good Behavior Chart

Behavior	Morning	Afternoon	Evening	Total
Follow Directions				
Listening				
Helping without being asked				
Respectfulness				
Kind to each other				
Good table manners				
Get ready in the morning without reminders				
Get ready in the evening without reminders				
Chores				
Homework				

The experts tell us that consistency is king, and we adhere to that with a religious fervor. We set routines in stone. We berate ourselves for inconsistencies and judge ourselves when our kids deviate from the plan. I hear from parents, "I know I need to be more consistent, but . . ."

But sometimes consistency isn't all it's cracked up to be. When we rigidly hold fast to routines and processes, we may miss when kids need:

- time to manage big emotions, even if it means being late.
- help to prioritize what's most important, especially after a long day at school.

- to stand next to their chair when they're feeling particularly hyperactive at dinner.

To effectively meet our kids where they are, they need us to recognize when we've asked enough for that day and relax on a system. To give them permission to start again fresh the next day.

The chart that worked best for my family was beyond simple: a blank points column for each child. When I caught them being good, I told them to give themselves points, which they could use to buy things. Bonus: they learned how to count to five using tally marks.

One of my favorite simple, flexible structures was allowing kids to choose homework locations. I was taught that kids should do homework at a desk, sitting up, head straight. I even had a tutor tilt my child's head back into place. It was ridiculously rigid. I bought into it because I didn't know any better.

Then I allowed my kids to decide on homework locations, with some negotiation. They did homework in forts and trees (always with one hand holding on), on porches and beds (horrors!). One kid's favorite spot was lying on the dining room table so she could bounce her foot off the side as a fidget. And you know what? They did their homework. That was the goal, right?

It's an art to motivate kids to use systems without overwhelm or pushback. So why make it too complicated? Embrace simplicity and flexibility. Stop allowing someone else's rigid structure to prevent your kids from achieving their goals.

Self-Talk: Solutions Are in the Successes

Before I started working only with adults and parents, I once coached a 14-year-old girl who wanted to do well in school but was struggling with homework. She was highly motivated by her social life, and I got curious when she told me she'd planned a sleepover. She explained every step of the process, including how she and her friends recruited parents to drive them. She proudly described a feat of executive function.

Planning a sleepover might sound frivolous, but once she understood the process she used to plan it, we were able to map her successes over to planning homework. Within minutes, she had a plan for drawing out her homework sequence on a piece of poster board to visualize the process as a reminder. Even better, it was all her idea.

Taylor-Klaus Points Chart

Tally Marks: 5 = ||||
MONTH:

Name:	Name:	Name:

PART TWO

Lean into what's working. How we do anything is how we do everything, so remember, success breeds success.

When my daughter became obsessed with solitaire, I thought it was distracting her from schoolwork. But when I stopped to look for successes, I realized she was playing to soothe her nerves (junior year of high school = stress!). Upon reflection, she realized that ordering simple things logically helped to get her brain organized, so her solitaire skills could translate to schoolwork. Solitaire helped her see a new possibility and paved the way for her to visually organize her homework planning in a new way.

> Lean into what's working. How we do anything is how we do everything, so remember, success breeds success.

Sometimes we feel like we're bouncing from one catastrophe to another without a moment to catch our breath. We gravitate to anything that reduces the chaos and helps us feel more on top of things. When the world offers dozens of opportunities to marinate in mistakes, it's tempting to learn only from what doesn't work. But that gets demoralizing, especially when kids take things personally and get defensive.

Instead it's liberating to focus on what they're doing well, no matter how small. Gems happen when we look for patterns, like a treasure map to find solutions for other challenges we might be facing. And it feels uplifting in the process.

Focusing on their successes is another way to play to kids' strengths, making them feel proud and good about themselves. They're much more likely to want more of *that* feeling than everything that makes them feel terrible. When kids feel success, it invites them to want more.

Kids may not be able to get their stuff together for school, for example, but if they can get it together for ultimate Frisbee practice (something they're motivated to do), then that can be a starting point.

Ask yourself, "What worked before?" Then apply those successes to a new scenario and repeat. This is another reason to keep things simple. We want kids to see clearly when they achieve success and identify what helps them achieve it.

Bottom line: Encourage your kid to focus on one thing at a time, feel really good about it, learn from it, and apply it to something new. And remember, your solutions are in your successes too. You just finished part 2 of this book! What worked that you can keep using in another arena?

Questions for Self-Discovery

- When have you focused on a solution as your goal? How did that work out?
- When have you focused on the process? What was different?
- What needs problem solving instead of fixing?
- Practice failing forward with the three magic questions to address a simple mistake. How does it help with your acceptance of the mistake?
- What processes do you want to focus on over outcomes?
- When do you make things complicated instead of simple?
- What successes could your child build on?

ARE YOU DROWNING IN INFORMATION OVERLOAD?

More than likely, you've spent months or years taking a "popcorn" approach to managing your kids' complex issues. If you're anything like me, you've bounced from one solution to another. You've searched for promises and bought the snake oil.

Maybe you've tried brain training, talk therapy, occupational therapy, vision therapy, nutritional therapy, remediation, special schools, tutoring, social skills classes, neuro-feedback, reward charts, behavior contracts, or all of the above. The list could go on and on. Parents of complex kids go to great lengths, doing everything in our power to help our kids.

And let's be clear—some of these approaches make a lot of sense as part of an overall strategy for supporting and treating your complex kids (except the snake oil). I do not for a minute mean to suggest that these therapies and support structures aren't useful—in many cases, they can be game-changing.

What I do want to communicate clearly is that when we start with these solutions, before we get a handle on what is happening and what is needed for our kids, it's like buying books for college before graduating from middle school.

It is absolutely essential to slow down, to get crystal clear on what challenges your child is facing, and create an incremental plan for action before speeding into piling one solution on top of another. You can't figure out what's working effectively if you're not clear on what you're trying to improve, and what your options are for doing just that.

This is where parenting with a coach approach provides an essential piece of the puzzle. I hope you'll let the Impact Model introduced in this section be your guide, step by step, to empower your child to reach their full potential.

Turning Information into Action

MAKING THIS WORK IN YOUR LIFE

If you skipped the first two sections of this book because you want to take action, please: go back to Part 2. Get the framework before you jump to action. Then, once you've learned about taking aim on a challenging situation, gathering information, and working through the four cornerstones, join me here to take action, rinse and repeat.

Parents tell me, "I've tried everything and nothing's worked." I walked in those shoes for more than a decade before I discovered that the key to success for my kids started with understanding, not solutions; it started with me, not them. Diving into quick fixes for a child's symptoms sacrifices effectiveness. It leads to wasted time, damaged relationships, and missed opportunities as children and teens become resistant to suggestions and refuse offers of help.

If children and teens don't gain self-awareness and skills to self-manage in high school, they likely won't turn to their parents for guidance when navigating the adult world.

According to all leading major medical associations (American Association of Pediatrics, the American Psychiatric Association, etc.), best practice treatment plans should provide support and training for parents. Still, most parents:

- routinely lack information about comprehensive treatment;
- are rarely directed to effective support to help them calm the chaos; and
- lack guidance to personalize treatment to their family's circumstances.

Many providers don't understand what's recommended by the term behavior therapy, nor the depth of what parents really need for help. Countless providers have told me they shy away from referring parents to behavioral supports because they don't want to offend parents and they fear the parents won't be receptive. It's kind of like a cardiologist not telling a patient to quit smoking because they just don't think they'll be compliant.

The old paradigm that all it takes to manage complex kids is a prescription and a star chart is just not true. If we want to effectively bring these kids into the process of self-management, we've got to understand their situation better, so that we can help them learn to manage it thoughtfully. We've got to enroll them to want to take action on their own behalf.

KARA'S STORY

Kara is upset because her daughter isn't obeying her rules. Frustrated, she put limits on her daughter's use of technology. In a public online forum, Kara wrote: "I'm a complete idiot for thinking my 14-year-old could handle a smart phone. Got it for her when she was 12, needed it for safety. Now all she does is sneak around and disobey me with it. It's going. She is getting a flip phone. I want so bad for her to be a normal teenager that can follow a simple rule around the phone. But her impulses are just too strong for her at this age. She's not mature enough to handle it." Kara is imposing rules without collaborating with her daughter, who doesn't see any reason to follow Kara's rules. When Kara understands that it's not "easy" for her daughter and works with her to find an effective solution, her daughter will be able to find the motivation to try to manage her impulsivity. As long as Kara is the only one who wants something to change, she's likely to be disappointed.

Bottom Line: "I want so badly for her to be a normal teenager who can follow a simple rule around the phone. But her impulses are just too strong for her at this age. She is not mature enough to handle it."

CHAPTER 11

"They Need to Be Able to Do This on Their Own"

Cultivating Ownership Gradually and Then Suddenly

"We all have the tendency to run into the future or go back into the past, to search for happiness elsewhere." —THICH NHAT HANH

Solving Their Problems without Them

Let's assume Kara established a reasonable rule for her daughter, such as "only use the phone after homework." Here's how it likely played out:

- Kara didn't like her daughter's phone usage, so she established a rule.
- Kara told her daughter the rule.
- Her daughter "disobeyed."
- Kara got frustrated and reacted on Facebook, "It's going."
- Kara told her daughter "it's going" because she can't handle simple rules.
- Her daughter freaked out, feeling misunderstood.

Chances are, Kara's daughter doesn't understand why her mom is making such a big deal, thinks her mom is unreasonable, wants to do things her way, and deep down feels her mother doesn't believe in her. Kara and her daughter both feel disempowered.

We're all guilty of this sometimes, myself included. We decide what's important for our kids, and then come up with solutions without their active participation. We tell them how we think they should do *their* stuff. Because they feel voiceless and powerless, they shut down, get defensive, or fight back. We hate it when people do this to us, and yet we do it to our kids.

It may be true that your child isn't independently handling homework, chores, or hygiene; engaging appropriately in class or with friends; or cleaning their room, starting homework, or turning it in. But the problem isn't that your kids aren't doing these things. The real problem is that you want them to do these things, and they don't truly see them as their agenda—yet. *You think* your kid has a problem, *you think* it needs to be addressed, and *you think* you know how they should handle it. So, *you decide* to help them "learn" to do it. Here's how it often plays out:

- You see what they need to do and how.
- You direct or convince them to do it.
- You give them a system to use.
- They don't use it.
- You get frustrated.
- You complain and make threats or give ultimatums.
- You start the cycle all over again.

It's hard for many of us to accept that your kids don't see whatever you think needs improvement as a problem. *Their* problem becomes that you think they have a problem (and want it fixed *your* way).

Kara sees the cell phone as a problem and wants her daughter to change her habits the way she thinks she should. Kara's daughter sees the problem differently: her mom is trying to control her. While Kara may be 100% correct, she needs to bring her daughter into the process for the dynamic to change.

WHOSE AGENDA AND SOLUTION IS IT?

It often backfires when we direct kids—especially older kids—to do basic tasks, such as homework, showering, or eating well. They get so desperate for control they'll "bite off their nose to spite their face." Even if it makes sense for them to study for that midterm, shower, or eat breakfast before school, they won't, just because you want them to.

Kids are generally unmotivated by doing things because it's good for them or because they "should." They need to have some skin in the game, a reason for changing their own behaviors—to have a reason to be part of the solution, not just feel like they are the problem. It either needs to be their agenda on some level or they need enough buy in to find motivation. If it's purely your agenda or solution, you're probably not setting up anyone for success.

Is your 9-year-old going to say, "Hey, Dad, I want to shower independently so you can take care of other things"? Not likely. But if they had a reason to make the effort, such as extra minutes of reading at bedtime, they might be willing to work with you to make it happen.

Coach's Reframe: A Collaborative Agenda

"I've learned so much—mostly that 90% of the problems we had were driven by us, not by our son. We had to understand how to help him learn to do what he was having trouble doing. Now, it's all him driving the process." —Diana, mother of a 19 year old

News flash: At the end of your life, you don't want to be the leading expert on your child. You want them to become the leading experts on themselves.

That's where the collaborative agenda comes in. They need you to help them figure themselves out, which is most effective when they see you as a support, not an obstacle. As you gradually transfer your knowledge to your kids, they'll come to believe they have the capacity to know themselves, eventually better than you do (even if they're not ready yet).

If I were Empress for a day, I would officially redefine parenting:

Parenting (noun) par·ent·ing | \ ʻper-ən-tiŋ \
The activity of compassionately collaborating with a child to foster effective problem-solving skills, so that the child is enrolled to achieve independence in adulthood to the greatest extent possible.

We want our kids to feel we're in this together and are on their team, that we've got their back, sharing the goal of **their** happiness and success. As Dr. Ross Greene's work emphasizes, collaboration is key to help kids take ownership of their lives and responsibilities. It's fundamental to teach them problem-solving skills, instead of feeling like they're problems for us to solve. "Why doesn't power work?" asked Greene in his 2019 keynote presentation. "Power causes conflict. Collaboration brings people together."

After years of directing kids through their lives, the shift to take a collaborative approach can be tough, because it requires:

- the patience of Job and the endurance of a marathon runner.
- letting go of our own agenda and supporting them in theirs.
- letting them do things their way, and giving them credit for their successes while guiding them to learn from mistakes.

With a collaborative approach, you help kids set goals and work to achieve them, instead of telling them what their goals should be. You help them discover what's important to them, so they can find a good reason to share your agenda—a reason besides "because I said so."

Encouraging kids to do things for themselves, not for you, empowers them. Learning. Grades. Making friends. Being kind. Even cleaning up the dinner dishes. (I know that's a stretch!) Those are ultimately *their* jobs, not just parent-pleasers. Do you want your child to do homework because they think it's important, or because you tell them to? To stay away from drugs because they want to be healthy and safe, or to avoid getting in trouble?

> Encouraging kids to do things for themselves, not for you, empowers them.

Around puberty, your child is going to lose the motivation to do things just to please you. But ideally, they'll always be motivated by what they want for themselves. That motivation lasts a lifetime. So if you want your kids to become independent adults, start gradually giving them autonomy and control much sooner. Help them see what *they're* responsible for, instead of seeing everything they do as a favor for you.

- If your child still needs you to be in parenting Phase 2 (see Chapter 4), start collaborating by getting their buy-in and giving them a voice in how (or when) they'll do something.
- If your child is ready for you to be in parenting Phase 3, give them ownership, empower them to assume responsibility, and offer support as needed.

Collaboration is about shared ownership and fostering independence, ultimately helping kids become fabulous human beings who will be motivated to "do the right thing" in life—such as *wanting* to take care of you when you're old. (Don't we all want that?)

THE FOUR PHASES OF PARENTING
Quick refresher (see Chapter 4).

Phase 1: Motivate effort and direct work. The child's agenda belongs to the parent, who provides appropriate motivation. Parents may get stuck here because it's familiar or they worry things won't get done.

Phase 2: Motivate ownership and model organization. Encourage kids to join you in planning. Guide kids through problem-solving and decision-making activities. When unsure, Phase 2 is a strong place to start.

Phase 3: Transfer ownership and support organization. Move into a support role. Ask permission to make suggestions and offer advice, empowering your teen's ownership and self-determination.

Phase 4: Empower, champion, and troubleshoot. Encourage your younger adults and offer problem-solving support as needed. Gradually move into adult relationships with kids, and remember a younger adult's brain development isn't completed until around age 25.

PART THREE

Strategy: Get Buy-In

When my kids were little and wanted to stay up late for something, my husband would call it "Rock 'n Roll Lifestyle." Instead of saying no, we would discuss our expectations if they stayed up late, such as waking up without being grumpy or going straight to bed and showering in the morning. We were transparent about the challenge, negotiating the decision and setting clear expectations. We didn't always say yes, but if we did, before agreeing our kids had to authentically buy in to the deal.

"Rock 'n Roll Lifestyle?" we'd ask.

"Rock 'n Roll Lifestyle," they'd reply.

"Shake on it?" we'd ask.

It was so cute when they'd shake their whole body!

It was a superb tool for getting buy-in. Not only did it save tons of stress, but the kids learned there are trade-offs in life. To get what they wanted, they had to make some agreements and understand natural consequences; afterwards, we'd discuss how it worked and whether it could happen again.

We still use "Rock 'n Roll Lifestyle" to this day, because it's a masterful structure to set clear expectations and get activated when we know something is likely to be stressful. One particularly early morning, I even overheard my husband saying "Rock 'n Roll Lifestyle" to himself in the mirror!

Leading people to take ownership of their lives is at the core of a collaborative approach. It starts to flow naturally when your child is driving the agenda (parenting Phase 3), but during much of our time as parents, our kids aren't fully ready for that. For many years, they need us to be parenting in or moving into Phase 2, relying heavily on getting their buy-in to try things, modify them, and try again.

Sometimes we gain buy-in through external factors, such as rewards, new experiences, or interest. And buy-in is even more powerful when it's grounded in intrinsic motivators, such as a sense of pride or accomplishment or feelings of success. If you "own" something, you're more likely to want to do it (or do it well), and you'll be willing to work at it. If you think you're doing it for someone else, why bother? Without buy-in, kids have no stake in a task. External motivators can help them get something done in the short term; internal motivators help them repeat it until they do it well.

My son tends to phone it in when he doesn't have buy-in on something, so for years I would say, "anything worth doing is worth doing well," hoping to plant a seed for when he was older. During his summer as a camp counselor, it bore fruit—he shared the message with his campers. He told me he didn't expect it to make a difference, but maybe it would help them in the future when there was something they really cared about. I appreciated the reminder that, even at camp, kids will phone it in when they don't have buy-in.

> Expecting blind obedience doesn't foster independence; teamwork with buy-in *does*.

Buy-in is essential for effective action. Kids need to have some reason to do what's being asked of them. If your kid doesn't care enough, it doesn't matter how good a system is. Before you start any action, make sure your child actually intends to use the plan you work on together. This goes for other members of the family too. If your child is on board but your spouse or a sibling is dismissive, that can undermine everything. Figure out what's in it for everyone.

The ultimate goal in parenting is to help your kids become independent and capable adults actively leading their own lives. Expecting blind obedience doesn't foster independence; teamwork with buy-in *does*.

Say No to Controlling

Well beyond the stereotypes of helicopter parents who do everything and boss everyone around, controlling happens in subtle ways. As parents, we become so expert at directing and controlling through every nuance of kids' lives that we don't realize we're doing it; it's almost like an occupational hazard.

But our need for control is at odds with our kids' growing need for autonomy. When we get stuck in control mode, we unwittingly sabotage their independence by:

- making things our agenda without exploring what's important to our kids;
- controlling little things, preventing our kids from practicing making decisions;
- ignoring buy-in to a goal or solution; and
- building resentment (theirs and ours), ultimately justifying their resistance.

One of the most insidious ways we control our kids is through language. Positive or negative, our words are powerful.

FIVE WAYS TO WATCH YOUR TONGUE

1. **Shift how you talk about your kids.** When we refer to our kids as "lazy" or "rude," it not only influences how others interpret their behaviors, it influences how we do. Choose nonjudgmental terms as you reference them, both to keep your focus on the positive and in case they overhear you from the other room!

2. **Change the language you use with your kids.** Many kids take things literally (especially younger kids, kids on the autism spectrum, or kids with language-processing disorders). Absolutes, such as "you never" and "I always have to," inadvertently lead to mistrust.

3. **Beware language that undermines ownership and buy in.**
Expressions such as "because I said so" and "it's for your own good"
unintentionally imply their responsibility is actually your agenda.
For example:

   - *"I need you to* get started on your homework." Whose
     agenda is it?
   - *"What do we have* for homework tonight?" Whose
     homework is it?
   - *"Can you do me a favor* and get started on your homework?"
     Is their homework a gift to you?

4. **Empower kids by encouraging them to be proud of themselves,**
instead of telling them how proud you are. Help them feel good for
themselves, not just to please you.

5. **Use code words to let go of control** and support emotional self-
regulation. Code words are cues to communicate succinctly, like a safe-
word or verbal short hand. The code word most of us know is *uncle*—a
word you call out when you've had enough. Collaborate to create code
words by agreeing on a behavior to improve. Get buy-in by letting your
kids do the naming.

How to Make Code Words Work

- Discuss the idea of code words and get agreement to give one a try.
- Agree on one behavior to change. Start simply—avoid the most
  volatile situation. Make sure your child wants to see change too.
- Let your child name the word you'll use (it's okay if it's ridiculous).
- Identify situations when it could be useful. Discuss who will use it,
  and for what reasons. Agree on what will happen when it is used.
- Practice with some role play or just talking through how it might work.
  Have fun and don't let it become a chore.
- Agree to a trial time. Three days? One week?
- Review and tweak as necessary ("Don't ever use that when I'm in the
  bath, Mom—then it won't work for me."). Give your child ownership to
  help you "fail forward." Learn from what works and what doesn't.

Here are some sample code words we used in our family:

- **Broccoli Ice Cream:** Someone is losing the ability to cope because they're hungry. Stop everything and get some food!
- **Bubble Gum:** Brace yourself, because you might not like what I'm about to tell you, but I've still got to tell you, okay? Let me know when you're ready for me to continue.
- **Basta:** It's fun until someone gets hurt, so we better stop now cause I'm about to lose it and I don't want Mom to stop us from playing.
- **Rope:** Back off, everyone—I'm trying really hard not to lose my cool.
- **Don't Poke the Bear:** Leave your sibling alone because they're not in a place to be messed with right now.
- **Do Stupid Smart:** I know you're going to make your own decisions, and I might not agree with what you're going to do, but please think it through and make sure you're not going to regret anything.

Say Yes to Connecting with A.C.E.

It's hard to know when we're on the right track. Parents frequently ask me, "Am I doing the right thing?" We want reassurance, to know we're making good decisions, to help our kids become independent. We need acknowledgment and compassion for the difficult road we're on. And so do our kids.

Remember when they were toddlers and they'd look at you after falling to see if they were hurt? It's similar now. There are so many upsets in a complex child's life, they still want you to kiss them and make them better, to trust their connection to you. They want to feel understood, listened to, heard. To know that you see and validate what's going on for them, acknowledging their hurt as real. As my husband, David Taylor-Klaus, often says, "being listened to feels so much like being loved, people can scarcely tell the difference."

In her video *The Difference Between Sympathy and Empathy*, Brené Brown explains Teresa Wiseman's research on the four qualities of empathy that "drive connection" with our kids:

1. Perspective taking
2. Staying out of judgment
3. Recognizing emotion in other people
4. Communicating that emotion

PART THREE

Says Brown, "What is empathy? And why is it very different from sympathy? Empathy fuels connection. Sympathy drives disconnection." For complex kids, connection is fundamental. As my kids have taught me again and again, "Mom, sometimes I just need you to say, 'poor baby.'"

When we're connected with our kids, we can engage with them, teach them, support them, empower them, and ultimately guide them to independence and success. When we're disconnected, they tune us out—shutting the door on open communication (if not slamming it in our faces). When they stop listening, it's like we hit our heads against that door, frustrated, scared, and clueless how to get them to open up.

The A.C.E. Method helps you communicate with connection.

Acknowledgment + Compassion = Empathy

Acknowledge: Verbalize what's going on for your child so they can recognize it. They'll feel heard instead of "wrong."

> *"Wow, when you were standing on the counter, I'm guessing you had forgotten that you're not supposed to do that, huh?"*

> *"When your sister's backpack knocked into you, it surprised you. I know you don't want to hurt her, and when you thought you were being hit, your instinct was to hit back."*

> *"When I asked you to take out the garbage, I'm wondering if you heard me or processed that I was asking you to do something."*

Compassion: Show that you understand how it feels to make a mistake or be asked to do something you don't want to do. For bonus points, use humor.

> *"When I'm really excited about something, it's hard for me to control myself too."*

> *"When I get startled, I get freaked out too, and sometimes I can't control myself. Remember when I saw that cockroach?"*

"When I'm concentrating on something, sometimes I don't realize someone is speaking to me."

Note: It helps to pause after A. and C. Maybe even repeat them a few times. When everyone's ready, move on to E.

Explore: Problem-solve how they might handle things differently in the future, negotiate a compromise, or create a code word. Allow your child to regain a sense of control. If they start getting upset, go back to A. and C.

"When you're trying to reach something high, would you ask for help or maybe use a step stool? What might remind you not to climb?"

"When you get startled, it can hurt people, even when you don't mean to. Let's think about how to help you respond differently when you get startled. I know you love your sister. Let's make sure she's okay and apologize, and then come up with new ideas. Sounds good?"

"When you're hyperfocused, it's like the rest of the world doesn't exist. I'll try to get your attention before I ask you to do something, okay? Should I tap your shoulder or ask for your attention?"

Self-Talk: Ask, Don't Tell

As my daughter backed out of the eighth-grade dance at the last minute, my husband questioned her about the choice she was making. Frustrated, she said, "I don't need a coach, I need a parent right now."

Smiling, her dad said, "go get in the car, you're going to the dance."

"I'll take a coach," she replied. She didn't end up going to the dance, but she understood her reasons for making that decision, and handled the friendship issue well—all with our full support.

Would I have preferred she go to the dance? Yes, actually. But she's an independent being with her own lessons to learn. Instead of fixating on what we thought she needed to do, we guided her to make a conscious, thoughtful decision about what she wanted to do. Could we have made her go to the dance? Certainly. But what would that have really accomplished? Sometimes we get so invested in teaching them what *we want* them to learn that we stand in the way of their learning what *they need* to learn.

As our kids get older, we need to heed the wisdom of Socrates and shift from telling to asking. With questions, kids learn to discover their own answers. We avoid "I told you so," empowering them to process information for themselves, develop the skills to figure things out, learn from experiences, and practice making decisions.

You might be "telling" too much if you hear yourself say things such as:

- "I tried to tell her that . . . "
- "I have already explained . . . "
- "I told them ..."
- "It's so important that . . . "
- "I need you to understand that . . . "
- "I made a list for him, but . . . "
- "I only have a few years left before . . . "
- "It's not okay if he . . . "

Asking questions is core to coaching. Not interrogations, but open-ended questions, generally without yes or no answers. Instead of telling people what to do or feel, questions guide people to think about what *they might do* or how *they actually feel.*

Questions are an invitation, a welcoming from one person to another. They say, "What you think, or say, or feel truly matters to me." Of course, it helps when we remember to listen for the answers.

> We get so invested in teaching them what *we want* them to learn that we stand in the way of their learning what *they need* to learn.

When most of our communication with our kids goes one way—when we're constantly trying to teach them, tell them, or convince them—communication breaks down. Eventually they stop listening altogether. Can you really blame them? It's human to resist feeling controlled.

Funny, when little kids want to do things by themselves, we proudly admire their independence and self-determination. We involve toddlers in decision making, giving them choices to avoid meltdowns.

The older they get, the more important that practice becomes, and yet somehow, we start lecturing more and giving fewer choices. Then they stop doing things just to please us, which is developmentally appropriate; it's an indication that they're developing a healthy sense of self. But we interpret that as a problem instead of an opportunity.

"But if they're not doing what they're supposed to, don't I have to make sure they get it done, or that they learn to do it?" you wonder.

> Help your child begin to see success as their responsibility.

The goal is to communicate so your child will actually receive information from you and be willing to do something with it.

It's our job to find teachable moments to educate our kids. We want to prepare them to step into the adult world, raise them with our values, and make sure they learn from our experiences. So I'm not suggesting that you stop giving directions or teaching your child.

The opportunity is to help your child begin to see success as their responsibility. Think about questions to help them focus on the next step. They might not choose the path you think is best (such as going to the school dance), but as they answer your questions, they'll develop their own agenda and step into ownership of their lives.

Questions for Self-Discovery

- When do you tend to solve your own problems, not your child's?
- How are you taking a collaborative approach?
- What helps you get your kids' buy-in?
- What are you trying too hard to control? You might want to journal on this one for a while.
- When can you imagine that using A.C.E. could be helpful for you? How do you think it will be helpful for your child?
- How comfortable are you with asking open-ended questions?

PART THREE

MY STORY

I started coaching when my youngest child was 6. Thankfully, as his emotional intensity peaked at age 9, I had learned to prioritize his emotional health over my need for him to "obey." As I practiced all of the tactics, strategies, and concepts offered in this book, we navigated his intense mood storms together, gradually finding a kind of détente. By the time he entered high school, meltdowns had given way to a wonderfully strong relationship, supported by his unusually excellent communication skills. At 18, he texted that he'd had a car accident just as I was stepping into a group-coaching call. I laughed out loud, took a deep breath, turned off my phone, and trusted that he had things under control. The text read: "Cops are on the way. Completely her fault. She feels really bad, though, so I'm being superfriendly. She called this 'the chillest car accident ever.' I'm having a fun time." Later he explained, "When the cop showed up, I turned down the music and told him that she gave me a love tap. He laughed. In fact, the only one I couldn't make laugh the whole time was the woman who hit me. She felt so bad, and I felt really bad for her."

Bottom Line: Stay the course, use the strategies, and trust the process. Your kid can become the extraordinary young adult they are destined to be. You'll get them there by standing beside them and moving forward together.

CHAPTER 12

"How Do I Know If It's Working?"

Bringing It All Together

> "We need to find the many small joys that life has to offer and help them grow." —THICH NHAT HANH

Even Conscious Parents Get Stuck

Imagine you're attending the circus, and a clown selects you from the crowd to join the act. You hesitate—the high wire? He whispers, "The bar is rigged to keep you balanced. You're safe." Reluctantly you agree. After all, this is just an act, there's a net for safety, and the fans are cheering wildly.

Parenting is a lot like that. It seems ridiculously risky and yet safe enough, all at the same time.

Parenting a complex child is like that too, with a twist. You're going along just fine and then suddenly, you watch in disbelief as the fans silently leave the tent and the circus performers disappear. You're afraid to look down to see if there's still a net. You think you're all alone on that high wire in the middle of the big tent, when you realize with horror that your child is on your shoulders. The only safety net for your child is you.

Before everything changed, surrounded by encouragement and confidence, you felt you were on a reasonably safe adventure. Now you feel stranded, compelled to find a safe landing for your child. It's not like you have a choice. You're out there on the wire: committed, terrified, feeling simultaneously responsible and irresponsible.

Your mission in this moment: get yourself and your child back to safety. How to do that, however, is muddy.

- At first you panic and scream for help; but that throws you off balance, so you take some deep breaths, regaining your center.
- Next you start inching toward the nearest landing, thinking you just need to move painfully slowly. You stop as you begin to wobble. That seemed like a good idea too.
- Now you're paralyzed, because you only know one thing for sure: you don't want to do anything that's not going to help. You're frozen.
- Desperate to get to the side, you try the other direction. Again, you teeter and stop with frustration. Now what?
- It dawns on you that you're embarrassed, even mortified. How did you end up in this situation? You don't want to need help, but you do.
- Finally, slowly, you take out your phone and call 911. The fire department brings a very tall ladder, secures the net, and gets you down to safety.
- When the ordeal is over, you feel like superman. Your child knows you're there for them every step of the way; that you'll get them through anything. They know that you've got this—and so do you!
- Suddenly you're back in the circus, surrounded by cheering fans, no longer on the high wire. Now, you're in a clown car, safe on the ground, appreciating the laughter, and having fun again.

Parents of complex kids try everything, again and again. Some of us panic. Some of us seek random help without a plan. Some of us try different things because they're right in front of us and seem like they should work (even if they don't). We do nothing because we're mortified, or because we don't know what to do. We get stuck because the fear of change is greater than the fear of the status quo, even when what we're doing isn't working.

I did all of that, for a dozen years. Like a pinball, I bounced from one specialist to another, screaming for help into a void. I was so afraid. I put my child in every therapy imaginable, trying to fix anything I could. I froze or picked up the slack. I enabled. I missed multiple chances to help my child learn how to learn, because I was doing everything possible to fix my kid.

It took a long time to get the help I really needed, help that would direct me to the most important truth of all: my kid only needs to trust that I've got them, and I'll figure it out. That, and I strongly prefer a clown car to the high wire!

Real change happens when we let go of resistance, shame, embarrassment, or whatever is holding us back, and ask for and accept the help we need. It may not be graceful. It may not be easy. It's most certainly not what we expected when we had kids. But it happens when you're willing to make a public spectacle of yourself, if necessary, and call for help, only to find out the answer is with you all along: trust yourself.

Coach's Reframe: Progress over Perfection (Rinse & Repeat)

During summer break, my son was hanging out with friends. He agreed to clean up the family room before I used it the next morning, assuring me he didn't need a reminder. When the room wasn't clean in the morning, I woke him. *"I'm really sorry I have to wake you, sweetie. I know you wanted to sleep in, but we had a deal that the family room would be ready this morning, and it's not. Please get up and clean up from last night."* He grumbled, mumbling something about doing it later. I stayed compassionate and clear. *"Seriously I know it stinks. Please, go clean out the room right now. My friends will be here soon."*

Was he happy about it? No, of course not. Was he grumpy while he was doing it? Yes, though not unreasonably rude. It was a natural consequence. He couldn't really argue with me, because I wasn't being unreasonable; I was holding him accountable to something he had previously agreed to. And I was doing it relatively nicely.

Before he used the room next, I reminded him to leave it so others could use it, and checked in on his plans to remember so he didn't get woken up again. No judgment, no shame. Just matter of fact. I haven't had to wake him up again (so far).

Dwight Eisenhower once wrote, "Plans are worthless, but planning is everything." This is particularly applicable to problem solving with complex kids. We shouldn't expect everything to work perfectly or go exactly as planned the first time we try it. Any efforts to improve our kids' self-management likely won't work the first (or second) time we try. Instead we want to remember that course correction is a normal part of the process.

In fact, endings and beginnings can get really blurry. Just when something gets comfortable, it changes again; and when you accomplish something, another challenge emerges. Every time you think you've learned what you need to know, there's something more for you to learn.

We tend to try things out of desperation or stick with something that's not working because we don't know what else to do. But there's incredible value in incremental progress. Step by step, we can guide our kids to self-awareness and independence, mostly in baby steps rather than giant leaps.

Rock climbing offers a wonderful metaphor for this. When climbing a rock face, a novice will stretch their arms as far as possible, pulling themselves up the wall; but they'll wear themselves out pretty quickly. An experienced climber knows that stamina and endurance come with baby steps. Spider climbing. Focusing on the feet, not the hands, looking for the next tiny increment of height to provide new opportunities within arm's reach.

> Incremental progress is actually what brings lasting change.

At the end of the day, incremental progress is actually what brings lasting change, rather than getting caught up in trying to make things perfect. Pause frequently to evaluate progress and make sure you're using your time and energy as effectively as possible. Diane and I like to call it *Rinse and Repeat*. It takes a few different forms:

- Stick with a solution, apply the magic three questions (see Chapter 10), tweak or improve it, and try again.
- Decide progress is good enough (see Chapter 8), and take aim at a new challenge.
- Recognize what's working and apply it to other challenges (see Chapter 10).
- Notice that what you thought was the problem is not actually the real problem, and start again with a new focus.

Pausing can be hard when you feel pressed, but it's essential. Pay attention to what's working and what's not. Whenever possible (or relevant), include your child in the conversation. Instead of shooting down kids' ideas, let them try something even if you're pretty sure it's not going to work (staying safe, of course). Then follow up without judgment to empower your child with Rinse & Repeat.

Strategy: Teach Kids to Ask for and Accept Help

"Sometimes I'm really good at asking for what I need, and other times I don't want to need help, and so I resist it. But I notice that every single time after I buck up and ask for the help I need, my life gets significantly easier, and brighter. It becomes easier to breathe. It becomes easier to walk. I want people to feel that, to experience the lightening of their load. Atlas held up the world all on his own, but we don't have to." —Bex Taylor-Klaus, *Flaunt Magazine*

Is there one strategy more important than anything else in this book? Yes.

In a sense, everything in this book is designed to encourage you to ask for the help you need and enroll your kids to ask for and accept help from you and from others. We want to develop kids' self-advocacy skills, helping them understand themselves and what they need, and learning to identify what will help them be successful. Although it's a difficult skill to transfer, it will profoundly support your kids throughout their lives.

Even though we've been acculturated to resist asking for help, no one does anything alone. We believe we should know how to help our kids, or that they'll grow out of it. We convince ourselves we just need to try harder, read one more book, hire a tutor, or—wait. Underneath it all, we don't want to need help from anyone.

Our kids feel the same way. Despite complex issues that make it difficult to manage their lives, they don't want to need help, from us or anyone. They feel they should be able to do what their peers can do, and they want to feel like everyone else. They avoid admitting they're struggling and resist help when it's offered to them. They want to believe they'll just grow out of it. Generally speaking, our kids resist help because they feel:

- it's not okay to make mistakes;
- it's not their agenda;
- they're unprepared for what's expected of them;
- they're unclear what help they need; and/or
- they're stressed but don't want anyone to know it.

It can be scary to ask for help; it requires vulnerability. There are so many complicated issues kids are navigating that it's hard to figure out whom to trust. Will they be met with openness and acceptance, rather than judgment or shame? Will it be worth the risk of embarrassment or shame? Will it really make a difference?

As we live in community with each other, we use help and allies in a whole host of ways. So, it's worth the effort to keep it casual and create an environment that makes it safe. If we really want our kids to accept help when we offer, we must model behavior and verbalize it often. Point out nonchalantly that most of us don't cut our own hair. Let them see you asking for help with your taxes and ask them for help with technology.

Staying connected with our kids allows them to trust us and, ultimately, to give themselves permission to ask for help, from us and others they trust. They'll learn to rely on relationships to seek help when they need it. Ultimately that will motivate them to seek guidance in years to come.

The ability to ask for help sets kids up for a lifetime of success. I experienced some of that success vicariously when my daughter called from college to say, "Mom, I went to talk to my dean to figure out that problem I was having." She was proud of herself, which is what I want most for her—to know that asking for help is what it takes to be successful.

Say No to Criticism

I took my kids on "dates," at least occasionally, when they were young, to have individual time with each of them. I gave myself two rules for those dates: let them choose the activity (within reason) and don't correct their behaviors (as long as they're safe). If they wanted to eat with their fingers, I would bite my tongue and focus on having fun.

Complex kids are constantly being redirected by friends, teachers, and parents. Half the time we don't realize we're doing it. It becomes natural to make simple corrections. But what we think of as a simple "no, try it this way" becomes larger than life to kids. They begin to hear every correction as a constant barrage of criticism.

"But I need to show them how to behave!" you object.

No, you actually don't. Not every time. Sometimes it's better to say nothing. More often than not, they know what they're supposed to do, but they can't quite get themselves to do it. They're already frustrated and don't need your reminder. Although it's unintentional on your part, rubbing mistakes in their face can make them want to stop trying.

> Staying connected with our kids allows them to trust us and, ultimately, to give themselves permission to ask for help, from us and others they trust.

You've probably heard about research that encourages us to praise kids three to five times for every one correction, to help build their self-esteem. Frankly that can be difficult to do, especially when we're not aware of how often we say things our kids hear as criticism. Their world is all about them, and they are wired to take things personally! So how do you come closer to the 5:1 ratio?

CATCH'EM BEING GOOD

My challenge to you: For one week avoid correcting your child in any way that's not essential. If it's dangerous, of course, keep them safe. Otherwise, see what happens when you keep their mistakes to yourself.

One week, avoid redirections. Notice what starts to change. While you're biting your tongue, enhance your little experiment by acknowledging anything you can and highlighting their sense of pride.

Thank them for everything you see them doing right, even if it's expected of them. It's amazing how far you can get with a simple "thanks for taking out the trash" or "that was a nice way of responding to your little brother." We all like to hear when we're doing a good job. More than likely, you won't overdo it. It's not easy to put a dent in the unconscious criticisms they hear daily, even when we're not saying anything. But it's definitely worth a shot.

Here are some things to try:

- Ask your child what she's proud of; acknowledge when you see it happen.
- When they do well, reinforce with, "I bet you feel good about that!"
- My favorite: "I bet you're really proud of yourself, aren't you?"
- Sometimes you can add, "Sure, I'm proud of you—that was awesome— but it's really cool that you're proud of yourself. *That's* really what's important, isn't it?!"

I know you might be breaking out in hives. You take your responsibility seriously, and you see it as your job to teach your kids to behave appropriately. I respect that, truly. And remember, there are lots of ways to teach any given topic. Our kids need a break from the "here's another lecture" method that many of us use as a default. When we focus on what's working, reinforcing their self-esteem and self-confidence, we'll gradually begin to notice that we don't need to lecture at all.

Consider giving it a try for a week: Limit your criticisms and critiques to the bare minimum, and focus on catching them being good instead. You might just notice it feels better for you as well.

Say Yes to Transparency

"We all put on masks. We all pretend to be something every day. I'm tired of it. I spent so long trying to be what they told me I had to be ... I just want to be me. And, I hope that by me being me, it'll inspire other kids to just be them. We need way more honesty, and transparency, and radical self-love in this world."
—Bex Taylor-Klaus, *Flaunt Magazine*

In an effort to improve my chronic lateness, I decided to stop making excuses. It might have been true that a slow truck was in front of me, there was traffic, or my driveway was blocked. But it was usually also true—truer—that I hadn't allowed enough time.

That's what I started to say when I arrived late. And you know what happened? Not only did people not noticeably judge or get offended, they responded with warmth, understanding, and grace. Most people were pleasantly surprised when I owned my truth.

This wasn't easy for me. As a perfectionist in recovery, I struggled with the idea that to be a good coach I had to come clean with my mistakes. I've always hated admitting mistakes! Transparency, a key concept in coaching, was difficult for me to put into practice. Being open, honest, straightforward, and authentic wasn't a struggle. But acknowledging mistakes without judgment, shame, or embarrassment? That was definitely a stretch.

> Transparency is about giving ourselves permission to be human, and, in doing so, giving everyone around us permission to do the same.

As an adult with undiagnosed learning and attention issues, easily embarrassed by anything short of perfection, I wanted to appear to have it all together, because on the inside it felt like things were falling apart. Maybe that's why I've waited until now to share this concept with you. This muscle takes time to build, and it can feel threatening. Fortunately many of the concepts covered throughout this book will help you get there.

Transparency is about giving ourselves permission to be human, and, in doing so, giving everyone around us permission to do the same.

Ironically transparency has actually become one of my superpowers, helping me connect with my kids, my clients, my family, and myself. It keeps me from taking things personally. I still resist it sometimes, but that's just part of it, isn't it?

Adults often feel like we're supposed to project a flawless image for children and teens. We keep mistakes to ourselves and avoid disagreeing in front of kids. We convince ourselves that modeling good behavior means modeling perfection, but the opposite is actually true.

Nobody likes perfect people, those who never make mistakes and can never be wrong. They're annoying. And they're particularly off-putting to kids, who are acutely aware of their own mistakes. Besides, kids love it when their parents admit to making mistakes! It makes us so much more approachable.

Preparing kids for real life as adults must include demonstrating that even amazing humans make mistakes; that even loving relationships have conflicts. When we hide truth from them, we're not doing them any favors.

To be truly human in all of its messiness is to make mistakes, learn from them, change our minds, be frustrated, and recover. If we only show kids shiny successes, they get an out-of-balance perspective and end up judging themselves harshly for typical human experiences. Transparency lets us give kids a glimpse into the full depth of who we are, without bringing them inappropriately into our adult problems. Simply put, it lets them know that adults have problems too.

Whether you're a teacher admitting you made a mistake in the wording of a test problem or a parent admitting you were out of line when you "lost it" at dinner, modeling transparency garners connection and respect. Kids feel there's someone real to trust and are more likely to engage and learn more effectively.

> We convince ourselves that modeling good behavior means modeling perfection, but the opposite is actually true.

Some of us are just as quirky as our kids. Allowing them to see that part of you gives them permission to be who they are. As I used to say to my kids whenever they'd get down on themselves for a mistake: "Permission to be human? Granted."

Self-Talk: Celebrate Unusual Victories

I was on a rare outing with my 10-year-old for a creek walk in a state park when I spotted the ugly, racist graffiti brightly painted on a rock's edge. Scraping away the letters KKK, I explained to my son why I found them offensive. We noticed uglier words on another rock. He searched for a small rock, climbed to the other boulder, and got to work. For hours we scraped and scratched, holding each other for safety, ignoring little scrapes and bruises. He never complained, owning clearly what was important about the task.

Despite the circumstances, I was grateful for a willing companion in doing the right thing. Teaching a valuable lesson without lecturing gave me the opportunity to bond with my son in a profound way. Together we modeled

> "Permission to be human? Granted."

responsible citizenship, and my son saw a glimmer of his own leadership. Later, walking toward our picnic spot, we passed an African American family with three small children heading toward the creek. My son smiled and said, "I'm glad those kids can go to the beach without being traumatized Mom."

The first "quick tip" that Diane and I published when ImpactADHD.com launched in 2011 was simple and straightforward: Celebrate!

Diane wrote, "Celebration is the act of honoring a person or event." Truly it's amazing how a simple concept such as celebration can turn the tide in the human experience, and in a child's development. Celebration as self-talk can inspire you to push through difficult moments that threaten to stop you in your tracks, not to mention what it can do for your relationship with your child. It feels great to praise someone you love, even for little things.

Because our kids internalize their frequent mistakes, their fear of disappointing us leads them to feel like we're pointing out mistakes when we're not. So celebrating hidden behavioral gems can counterbalance their constant sense of feeling "wrong," promoting positive self-esteem.

Extend celebrations beyond standard birthdays and holidays to include less traditional victories—even silver-linings in difficult experiences, such as when we encountered the graffiti. These approaches offer an enormous payoff:

1. **Celebrate the small stuff.** Find something in your child's life to honor every day and imagine there's no success too small to celebrate. Let loose and have fun; get silly and throw random dance parties. It may be embarrassing for kids in the short term, but later on they'll catch themselves smiling at the memory of the "nagging" mother or "disapproving" father singing into a kitchen spoon!

2. **Look for the victories in mistakes.** When things aren't going so well, look for little victories and celebrate the successes in them:

   - Your child is not being productive while doing homework? Say something positive about the effort.
   - Your kid cleared the plate to the sink but not the dishwasher? Acknowledge them for clearing the plate.

- Your kid finished homework with no time to spare? Congratulate them for getting it done!

3. **Find the silver lining wherever you can.** Sometimes the celebration we need most is not an obvious "happy" thing but a silver lining in a difficult time. We start our group-coaching calls with celebrations, such as mornings going smoothly, homework getting turned in, or kids getting off technology without a fight. But they also celebrate that they made it to the call, that they didn't lose their cool when their child behaved rudely, or that they were having good conversations even though their teen is failing classes. Sometimes our celebrations are hidden in what we might have once considered a crisis.

Celebrations don't have to be limited to external achievements and milestones; instead embrace the daily habit of looking for small, unusual, hidden treasures. Celebration is about what we choose to look for and see, how we respond to how our kids are behaving in different situations, and how we manage our expectations.

Celebration is at the core of the coach approach. It's fundamental to how we communicate with our kids. And ultimately, it's about how we share the load and transfer the baton. Because raising complex kids is humbling. It's daunting. It's unbelievably frustrating. And when you embrace it—for all its trials and tribulations—it can bring you more joy than anything you've even imagined possible in your entire life.

Are you ready to enjoy the ride?

Questions for Self-Discovery

- When and how do you get stuck?
- When have you found success in tweaking and trying again?
- How are your kids about asking for help? What about you?
- When do you catch your kids being good?
- How can transparency help you connect with your kids?
- What small or hidden victories will you celebrate?

AFTERWORD

A Letter from Elaine and Diane

"The way to understanding is first to listen to yourself." —THICH NHAT HANH

Dear Parents and Professionals,

When we started ImpactADHD.com back in 2011, ImpactParents.com, there was plenty of support available for complex kids but virtually nothing available to help the adults who were raising them. When we became coaches, we became much better parents to our complex kids, and it wasn't rocket science. We realized it was something we could teach to other parents. We knew from experience that parents don't need lectures or therapy. Instead they need real guidance and support, so that they can provide the help their kids need most.

We stepped in to fill a clear gap in services. Coaching had not been available to us when our kids were younger. And we knew from our own experience and that of our clients that parents can make a world of difference in the lives of their kids. In no time we expanded to include teachers in the conversation, because they were struggling with the same problems. The experts were telling everyone *what* to do, but no one was helping them figure out *how* to do it.

This book captures the foundational concepts, strategies, tips, and tricks that we've borrowed from the world of coaching to teach parents and educators *how* to effectively support the complex kids in their lives. It's just a beginning. Most people need more than ideas and information; they need a combination of training, coaching, and support to really get a handle on what's involved with raising complex kids. While these kids aren't easy to raise or educate, chances are your experience is not as unusual as you believe, and this will start you on the path to more confidence and calm.

We want to remind you that you're not alone. It's normal to feel over-whelmed, frustrated, or whatever it is you're feeling. It's normal to yell or control or avoid or feel lost. And just when you feel like you've got a handle on things, they'll change again—that's normal too.

And we want to remind you that you can make a huge difference. There are lots of ways to get the support you need, and it's up to you to ask for it. We can help you take the information in this book and put it into practice, if you choose to reach out to us for help. Whether it's with us or somewhere else, we want to encourage you to ask for and accept help—and teach your kids to do the same.

What we want for you—for all parents—is to help you build a strong, connected relationship with your kids, so that you can help them build a strong, connected relationship with themselves.

And most of all, we want to remind you of something that you may forget from time to time: You've got this!

Elaine Taylor-Klaus & Diane Dempster
Cofounders of ImpactParents.com
Creators of and SanitySchool.com

Discussion Group Guide

The Essential Guide to Raising Complex Kids is structured so that parents and professionals can use it in group discussions. Questions at the end of each chapter and below were developed to guide book-club discussion groups, parent discussions at your child's school, faculty in-service workshops, community center support groups, or individuals while reading the book. Certified trainers from Sanity School® may also be available to provide onsite assistance.

Although *The Essential Guide to Raising Complex Kids* stands on its own as a framework for raising and educating complex kids using a coach approach, it was also created to accompany the Sanity School® behavior-therapy training program for parents or teachers. Groups can be convened to watch the virtual trainings together or independently, followed by group discussion. Sanity School is available virtually on demand, with in-person trainings offered by certified trainers in specific locations globally.

Ideally these questions could be broken up into six sessions.

Session 1: Raising Complex Kids with a Coach Approach
Chapters 1–6

Questions about children/teens:
- How can letting go lead you to parent or teach from inspiration?
- What could a fresh start look like for you, starting now?
- Discuss how strengthening relationships, with yourself and your family or class, can improve things for your child or students.
- What interferes with your relationships (e.g., judgment, blame, resentment, etc.)?
- Which of the four parenting phases do you typically see yourself in? Where does your child need you to be more often? Your students?
- Discuss the value of taking aim very specifically compared to taking aim on general problems.
- Where do shame and blame interfere with your ability to support your child/students?
- Discuss forgiveness. Who wants or needs forgiveness? From whom?
- In what ways are you a "good fit" for your quirky child/students? How are you not?

- Discuss naughty vs. neurological in the context of taking a disability perspective.

Questions about adult self-care:
- What would be helpful for you to accept?
- What would it mean for you to put the stick down?
- When are you really putting on your oxygen mask first? When are you not?
- Discuss how strengthening relationships can improve your life.
- What gremlin messages keep you from feeling confident?
- What's the potential benefit of pacing yourself for the marathon, as it relates to your parenting or teaching?
- What's important to you?
- Discuss the difference between responding and reacting.

Session 2: Activating the Brain *Chapter 7*

Questions about children/teens:
- What's important about activating the brain?
- Discuss the six aspects of executive function.
- Discuss the role of motivation for complex kids.
- What's the value of ownership for complex kids?
- How are you thinking differently about the use of rewards?

Questions about adult self-care:
- In what ways do you tend to catastrophize? Discuss.
- How do you currently manage your own triggers?
- What feeds you?
- When do you most need to activate your brain, and what are some ways that you do that?

Session 3: Positivity *Chapter 8*

Questions about children/teens:
- What will kids/students remember about the tone of your home/ classroom in twenty years?
- In what ways do you (or can you) play to your child's/students' strengths?
- How are you unintentionally setting expectations of perfection?
- What are the obstacles and opportunities to make it okay to make mistakes?

Questions about adult self-care:
- How do you connect with your child/students?
- How is perfectionism impacting your life?
- How can you apply radical compassion to yourself?

Session 4: Shifting Expectations *Chapter 9*

Questions about children/teens:
- How does your child/student struggle because of unrealistic expectations?
- What stands in the way of you meeting kids/students where they are?
- Discuss the relationship between consequences and punishment.
- Discuss the potential impact of assuming best intentions on your child/students.

Questions about adult self-care:
- How are you setting unrealistic expectations for yourself?
- How can assuming best intentions support you?
- Who are your greatest champions?

Session 5: Using Systems and Structures *Chapter 10*

Questions about children/teens:
- Discuss the difference between fixing and problem solving.
- How are you focusing on results at the expense of the process?
- What's the impact of making things too complicated or rigid?
- Discuss how successes can lead to solutions in other areas.

Questions about adult self-care:
- What are your challenges with failing forward?
- What's the value to you of keeping things simple and flexible?
- Share and celebrate recent successes in putting yourself back on your list.

Session 6: Putting It All Together *Chapters 11–12*

Questions about children/teens:
- What's the value of a collaborative agenda?
- Discuss the opportunities for and challenges of getting buy-in.
- Discuss how language can empower kids to take ownership.
- What opportunities do you see in using A.C.E.?
- Discuss the value of kids/students learning from questions instead of beind directed.
- When are you "telling" when you could be "asking"?
- Why is asking for and accepting help such an important life skill?
- Discuss the reasons your kids/students resist asking for or accepting help.
- How do you catch your kids/students being good?
- Discuss the value of adult transparency for children and teens.

Questions about adult self-care:
- Why is asking for and accepting help important for you?
- Brainstorm potential behaviors when code words that could be useful for you.
- How can a focus on progress over perfection support you?
- How can transparency take pressure off of you?
- What unusual victories can you celebrate?

Resources

The best resources for parents and educators are those that are trusted to be effective, wellinformed, easily accessible, and applicable to your needs. When possible, they should be reinforced with support. To make sure you avoid broken links or wild goose chases, I'm making all additional resources available for you on ImpactParents.com.

ImpactParents.com is a free, public-service content website with an award-winning blog. Its resources are regularly updated. You'll find references mentioned throughout the book, plus others that Diane and I or the members of our community trust most. All resources and book recommendations are vetted or reviewed by us or our members. If you can't find what or who you're looking for, email TheTeam@ImpactParents.com and ask for help. If you have other nationally or internationally accessible resources you'd like to suggest, please send them for our review and possible inclusion.

Resources for Parents

Free Materials on ImpactParents.com

impactparents.com/start-here

impactparents.com/resources/free-impactparents-resources-for-parents/

ImpactParents Support Products and Programs

impactparents.com/online-store

Recommended Reading Carousel

impactparents.com/resources/recommended-reading/

Trusted Colleagues and Organizations

impactparents.com/resources/friends-of-impactparents/

Resources for Professionals

ImpactParents Professional Training and Certification Programs

impactparents.com/for-professionals/

Trusted Colleagues and Organizations

impactparents.com/resources/friends-of-impactparents/

To Support the free resources made available by ImpactParents.com, please go to impactparents.com/patreon

A Note about Recommended Treatment and Behavior Therapy

Regardless of what makes a child complex, adults are part of their recommended treatment. It doesn't matter what chronic condition a child has—ADHD, anxiety, juvenile diabetes, or obesity, for example—when medication, remediation, or behavior changes are recommended to manage a child's particular challenges, behavior-therapy training provides essential support for adults to help kids learn to manage themselves.

Behavior therapy is a confusing term. According to the CDC website, "Parent Training in Behavior Therapy is also known as Behavior Management Training for Parents, Parent Behavior Therapy, Behavioral Parent Training, or just Parent Training." According to HealthyChildren.org, "There are many forms of behavior therapy, but all have a common goal—to change the child's physical and social environments to help the child improve [their] behavior." No matter how you define behavior therapy, its purpose is clear: to create environments in a child's life so that the child can "learn or strengthen positive behaviors and eliminate unwanted or problem behaviors." (CDC).

Whether done in classes, groups, or private sessions, parent or teacher training in behavior therapy should help adults learn how to "better understand their child's behavioral issues and learn . . . skills specific to these problems" (CDC). Training in behavior management is generally provided by coaches, educational therapists, counselors, psychologists, and social workers. Sometimes professionals are trained to provide behavior therapy directly to children, which may bypass the important role of parent education.

In my opinion, one of the best (and often most affordable) options is working with a parent coach. Because anyone can "call themselves" a coach, it is important to select professionals who adhere to established professional standards and ethical guidelines. Additional training is also recommended for working with families or teachers whose children have complex needs. A parent coach should be certified by the International Coach Federation (ICF) and well educated about the range of conditions facing complex families. Many parent coaches work on the phone or video, significantly reducing costs and increasing access to services. When location is not a limiting factor, parents can get support at a time that works for their schedule, without having to drive long distances.

Acknowledgments

I understand why authors retreat to secluded cabins. Writing is an obsessive experience you don't want to impose on anyone. And yet, as a mom, wife, CEO, coach, daughter, and friend, I wrote this book in all my free time (cue laughter). I want to acknowledge absolutely everyone who came in contact with me over the year(s) who may have found me a single-minded companion. I was. I appreciate your generosity, kindness, and grace.

Special thanks:

Jim at LGRLiterary for seeing my vision, and Quarto, for making it reality. Jeff, for capturing the essence of our parenting archetypes. And Ned, for your beautiful prose.

My amazing team at ImpactADHD.com, for your encouragement and enthusiasm. Diane, Natasha, Shelley, Brit, Jeremy, Claire, Caitlin, Hilary—Monday meetings start the week with a smile, which is truly something to celebrate.

My spectacular parenting tribe, clients and community around the globe—your vulnerability, transparency, and trust are humbling and empowering. We love supporting you each day. You make a difference!

My home crew— Shelley, for creating space and being my cheerleader; Suzie, for more than a decade of just everything; Sarah, for keeping home and office habitable; Sophie, for ever-presence and puppy love.

My parents (Mom, Dad, Mom), my most authentic cheerleaders.

My dear friends, siblings, and neighbors—and all your amazing kids— for a deep sense of connection and belonging, even in my absence.

Diane, after nearly a decade of conscious partnership, I cannot imagine my world without you. I hope I've done you proud, represented our work honorably. Your wisdom shines through the pages.

My kids, Bex & Alicia, Syd, Josh—my puppies— you're my muses, my joy, why I do this amazing work in the world. Thanks for your patience, for allowing me to share your stories in service, and for seeing the gifts in your challenges.

My champion and partner, David Taylor-Klaus. I love getting to share this work with you, birthing books, our open nest—and I love you.

My coaching community: I am complete, for now.

About the Author

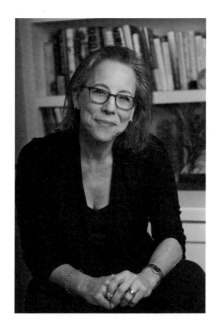

Since she was a teenager, Elaine Taylor-Klaus, PCC, only ever wanted to change the world; now, as an author, adult educator, and certified coach, she is doing just that. A trailblazing advocate for parents of complex kids, Elaine co-founded the ground-breaking ImpactADHD.com in 2011 to provide coaching, training and support for parents who were struggling to raise kids facing challenges with life and learning.

ImpactADHD's innovations and blog have earned awards and accolades, and their programs, based on the innovative Impact Model, offer perspective, practical skills, and hope—so that parents can raise children and teens with confidence and calm. Elaine co-created the Sanity School® behavior therapy training program, which serves thousands of parents and teachers around the globe, both online and delivered by licensed providers in local communities from Alaska to Melbourne. Internationally recognized as a voice for empowering parents when raising kids in complex circumstances, Elaine loves to travel and speak at schools and conferences. Her previous books include *Live Like You're Doing It on Purpose: Three Secrets to a Happy Life* and *Parenting ADHD Now! Easy Intervention Strategies to Empower Kids with ADHD* and she's been featured in numerous anthologies.

She is married to David Taylor-Klaus of DTK Coaching. Together they raised three complex kids and now enjoy parenting four young adults, two dogs, and a granddog.

Index

190

First Published in 2020 by Fair Winds Press,
an imprint of The Quarto Group,
100 Cummings Center, Suite 265-D
Beverly, MA 01915, USA.
T (978) 282-9590 F (978) 283-2742
QuartoKnows.com

Fair Winds Press titles are also available at discount for retail, wholesale, promotional, and bulk purchase. For details, contact the Special Sales Manager by email at specialsales@quarto.com or by mail at The Quarto Group, Attn: Special Sales Manager, 100 Cummings Center, Suite 265-D, Beverly, MA 01915, USA.

24 23 22 21 20   1 2 3 4 5

ISBN: 978-1-59233-935-8

Digital edition published in 2020

Library of Congress Cataloging-in-Publication Data

Names: Taylor-Klaud, Elaine, author.
Title: The essential guide to raising complex kids with ADHD, anxiety, and
    more : what parents and teachers really need to know to empower
    complicated kids with confidence and calm /
Elaine Taylor-Klaud, PCC,
    CPCC.
Description: Beverly, MA : Fair Winds Press, [2020] | Includes index. |
    Summary: "The Essential Guide to Raising Complex Kids is a step-by-step
    guide and coaching book for parents raising kids with ADHD, anxiety, and
    other challenges, written by renowned ADHD educator Elaine
    Taylor-Klaus"-- Provided by publisher.
Identifiers: LCCN 2020012692 | ISBN 9781592339358 (trade paperback) | ISBN
    9781631598449 (ebook)
Subjects: LCSH: Attention-deficit hyperactivity disorder--Popular works. |
    Anxiety in children--Popular works. | Behavior disorders in
    children--Popular works. | Child rearing--Popular works.
Classification: LCC RJ506.H9 T39 2020 | DDC 618.92/8589--dc23
LC record available at https://lccn.loc.gov/2020012692

Design: Debbie Berne
Illustration: Jeffrey Alan Gregory

Printed in China

ImpactADHD® and Sanity School® are registered trademarks of Diane Dempster and Elaine Taylor-Klaus.